CHAPTER 6   SPECIMEN CONSIDERATIONS AND SPECIAL PROCEDURES 195

THE COMPLETE TEXTBOOK OF PHLEBOTOMY,

2nd Edition

To my wife and family, who encourage and
support me when I am in my book-writing mode.
To all my students and staff, who keep challenging
me to do it better and reach for quality and
customer service in all that is done.

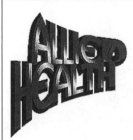

THE COMPLETE TEXTBOOK OF PHLEBOTOMY,

2nd Edition

Lynn B. Hoeltke, M.B.A., M.T. (A.S.C.P.), P.B.T., D.L.M.

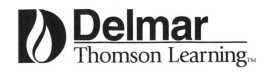

Africa • Australia • Canada • Denmark • Japan • Mexico • New Zealand • Philippines
Puerto Rico • Singapore • Spain • United Kingdom • United States

Cover Design: Jay Purcell

Delmar Staff:

Business Unit Director: William Brottmiller
Executive Editor: Cathy L. Esperti
Developmental Editor: Jill Rembetski
Executive Marketing Manager: Dawn F. Gerrain

Channel Manager: Nicole L. Benson
Project Editor: Patricia Gillivan
Production Coordinator: John Mickelbank
Art/Design Coordinator: Jay Purcell

For more information, contact Delmar, 3 Columbia Circle, PO Box 15015, Albany, NY 12212-0515; or find us on the World Wide Web at http://www.delmar.com

Asia
Thomson Learning
60 Albert Street, #15-01
Albert Complex
Singapore 189969
Tel: 65 336 6411
Fax: 65 336 7411
Japan:
Thomson Learning
Palaceside Building 5F
1-1-1 Hitotsubashi, Chiyoda-ku
Tokyo 100 0003 Japan
Tel: 813 5218 6544
Fax: 813 5218 6551
Australia/New Zealand:
Nelson/Thomson Learning
102 Dodds Street
South Melbourne, Victoria 3205
Australia
Tel: 61 39 685 4111
Fax: 61 39 685 4199

UK/Europe/Middle East
Thomson Learning
Berkshire House
168-173 High Holborn
London
WC1V 7AA United Kingdom
Tel: 44 171 497 1422
Fax: 44 171 497 1426
Thomas Nelson & Sons LTD
Nelson House
Mayfield Road
Walton-on-Thames
KT 12 5PL United Kingdom
Tel: 44 1932 2522111
Fax: 44 1932 246574
Latin America:
Thomson Learning
Seneca, 53
Colonia Polanco
11560 Mexico D.F. Mexico
Tel: 525-281-2906
Fax: 525-281-2656

Canada:
Nelson/Thomson Learning
1120 Birchmount Road
Scarborough, Ontario
Canada M1K 5G4
Tel: 416-752-9100
Fax: 416-752-8102
Spain:
Thomson Learning
Calle Magallanes, 25
28015-MADRID
ESPANA
Tel: 34 91 446 33 50
Fax: 34 91 445 62 18
International Headquarters:
Thomson Learning
International Division
290 Harbor Drive, 2nd Floor
Stamford, CT 06902-7477
Tel: 203-969-8700
Fax: 203-969-8751

Library of Congress Cataloging-in-Publication Data
Hoeltke, Lynn B.
    The complete textbook of phlebotomy / Lynn B. Hoeltke. — 2nd ed.
        p.   cm.
    Includes bibliographical references and index.
    ISBN 0-7668-0927-7
    1. Phlebotomy. I. Title.
    [DNLM: 1. Phlebotomy—methods. WB 381 H694c 2000]
RM182.H64 2000
616.07'561—dc21
DNLM/DLC
for Library of Congress   99-36290
                                                                CIP

TABLE OF CONTENTS

LIST OF PROCEDURES

PREFACE

There are several books on the market about phlebotomy. This book takes a different approach than many other texts, in that it strongly emphasizes a hands-on approach to learning the skills and knowledge needed to become the multiskilled professional needed in the 21st century. The individuals who will find this book useful are students wishing to learn phlebotomy for a career, medical assistants needing phlebotomy skills to work in a physician's office, and hospital nurses who are expected to perform phlebotomy in addition to their other duties.

Traditionally, the task of phlebotomy was centralized in the clinical laboratory. The task of phlebotomy is now decentralized and performed by many types of multiskilled individuals. These individuals will often not be at or near a hospital. They will be in physician offices, clinics, or laboratory-operated outpatient settings. These outpatient patient service centers (PSCs) are a new focus in the core laboratory concept.

In writing this book, I have used national standards to establish criteria for the proper collection of blood specimens. The National Committee for Clinical Laboratory Standards (NCCLS) and the *Federal Register* detailing Occupational Safety and Health Administration (OSHA) rules and regulations are the primary sources for establishing proper procedures. Health care centers follow these standards and regulations. By following them and by better knowing the importance of proper specimen collection, we will provide patients with the highest quality care available. Developing the phlebotomist's ability to improve patient care is the main purpose of this book.

Phlebotomy is an invasive procedure that requires a depth of knowledge and an ability to provide the most accurate and risk-free technique in the collection of a blood sample. The knowledge gained from this book is more than just the ability to collect a blood sample. The reader will have a better knowledge of what is in the blood sample and why the blood sample was collected.

HOW THE TEXT IS ORGANIZED

The Complete Textbook of Phlebotomy, 2nd Edition presents complete, in-depth training in the skills and knowledge needed for today's multiskilled phlebotomist. The chapters are arranged in a logical flow to develop the reader's knowledge. As the world of health care becomes more complex, the book covers these more complex elements. The areas covered are

- Introduction to Phlebotomy
- Safety in Phlebotomy
- Phlebotomy Equipment
- Phlebotomy Technique
- The Challenge of Phlebotomy
- Special Considerations and Special Procedures
- Customer Service
- Compliance
- Competency
- Appendix of Frequently Ordered Lab Tests
- Glossary

HOW EACH CHAPTER IS ORGANIZED

All chapters contain similar features and are arranged to highlight key points needed in the phlebotomy education process. The logical flow of the chapters helps the reader develop and build knowledge as each chapter is completed. Each chapter contains

- Objectives
- A list of key terms
- Graphic icons, tables and figures
- Procedures with step-by-step instructions
- Review questions
- Critical thinking questions

NEW TO THIS SECOND EDITION

This second edition has been updated and expanded throughout. A color insert has been added to emphasize illustrations and photographs that are best shown with color. The last three chapters are new to this type of textbook. These chapters cover the three "C's" of phlebotomy: customer service, compliance, and competency. Even after gaining the ability to collect a blood sample, each phlebotomist must know how to please the customer, know how to be legally correct in what is done, and be able to document his or her knowledge and ability to do the task correctly.

INSTRUCTOR'S GUIDE

A comprehensive instructor's guide is available. The guide includes answers for all review questions, and answers and explanations for all critical thinking questions. In addition to providing information from the textbook, the instructor's guide provides outlines on how to teach phlebotomy to all levels of students, from technical college students to experienced nursing staff. A competency training guide is also included to help in documenting the competency of a new phlebotomist in the workplace. For the individual wishing to obtain a national certification, a list of test questions and answers are included to use as a practice test.

ABOUT THE AUTHOR

Lynn B. Hoeltke, M.B.A., M.T. (A.S.C.P.), P.B.T., D.L.M., is the director of patient service centers for a leading joint venture laboratory in the Midwest. He has thirty years' experience in various laboratory leadership roles. He directs twelve patient service center sites and is also a faculty member teaching phlebotomy at IVY Tech State College. He has developed and taught a nursing-based phlebotomy program for a hospital. He has consulted with several nursing homes and laboratories in teaching phlebotomy techniques to their staff. He has published several magazine articles, been a contributing author for *Comprehensive Medical Assisting*, and is author of *The Clinical Laboratory Manual Series: Phlebotomy*, both by Delmar.

ACKNOWLEDGMENTS

The following reviewers assisted in the revision of this new edition: Judith D. Bennett, C.M.A., R.M.A., R.P.T., Applied Career Training, The Allied Health School, Arlington, VA; Richard N. Coffey, M.T. (A.S.C.P.), Freeport Memorial Hospital, Freeport, IL; Diane M. Klieger, R.N., M.B.A., C.M.A., Program Director,

Medical Assisting, Pinellas Technical Education Centers (PTEC), St. Petersburg, FL; Tese Gorszwick, M.T. (A.S.C.P.) C.P.T. (A.S.P.T.), Medical Laboratory Assistant/Phlebotomy Program, Oceanside Unified School District, Oceanside, CA; Jan Meitl, M.T. (A.S.C.P.), Director, Medical Assistant Program, Topeka Technical College, Topeka, KS; Barbara L. Stein, M.S., M.T. (A.S.C.P.) S.H., C.M.A., Retired, Program Director, Medical Assisting, Bryant & Stratton, Rochester, NY; and Mariel York, M.A., C.M.A., Medical Assisting, Applied Career Training, Alexandria, VA.

Chapter 1

INTRODUCTION TO PHLEBOTOMY

O B J E C T I V E S

After studying this chapter, you should be able to:

1. Explain why blood is collected by the phlebotomist today.
2. Outline the phlebotomist's responsibilities to the patient.
3. Explain why the phlebotomist has a special responsibility to present a neat, pleasant, and competent **demeanor.**
4. Identify departments within the hospital, and explain their function.
5. Identify each section of the laboratory.
6. Identify members of the laboratory staff.
7. Describe the importance of communication within the laboratory and with other departments of the hospital.
8. Define ethics.
9. List five patient rights.
10. Explain advance directives.
11. Describe the characteristics of the different types of blood cells.

12. Describe the major difference between the walls of the arteries and the walls of the veins.
13. Differentiate between serum and plasma.
14. Name the parts of the heart, and describe their function.
15. Trace the flow of blood through the heart.
16. Locate the veins in the arm.
17. Explain systolic and diastolic pressure.
18. Explain the conductive system of the heart.
19. Explain the purpose of the lymph system.

KEY TERMS

Advance Directive	Document stipulating the kind of life-prolonging medical care permitted for a patient.
Anticoagulant	A chemical substance that prevents the blood from clotting.
Buffy Coat	A layer of cells in an anticoagulant tube of blood that is positioned between the red blood cells and the plasma layers. The buffy coat consists of white blood cells and platelets.
Centrifuge	An instrument that spins and separates blood into layers depending on the weight of the layer. The heavier elements are pushed to the bottom due to centrifical force.
Compatible	Substances that can be mixed without reacting with one another.
Demeanor	The outward behavior of an individual.
Diastolic	Blood pressure when the heart is at rest.
Endocarditis	Infection of the inner membrane layer of the heart.
Erythrocytes	Also known as red blood cells.
Esoteric	Laboratory tests that are not commonly done. These tests are usually sent to another laboratory that specializes in a specific test.
Ethics	Professional code of conduct in treatment of patients.
Hemopoiesis	Formation of blood cells.

Leukocytes	Also known as white blood cells.
Occluded	Blocked, preventing a normal flow of blood.
Pathology	Study of the nature and cause of disease.
Phlebotomy	Act or practice of bloodletting as a therapeutic or diagnostic measure.
Plasma	Fluid portion of the blood when no clotting has taken place.
Serum	Fluid portion of the blood after clotting has taken place.
Systolic	Blood pressure when the heart is fully contracted.
Thrombocytes	Also known as platelets.
Venipuncture	Collection of blood from a vein by penetrating the vein with a needle.

HISTORY OF PHLEBOTOMY

Phlebotomy is the process of collecting blood and is defined in Webster's dictionary as "the act or practice of bloodletting as a therapeutic measure." The history of bloodletting dates back to the early Egyptians and continues into modern times. It was once thought the practice would rid the body of diseases and provide a cure-all for almost all ailments. Picture a Roman gladiator bleeding and being carried off on a stretcher to receive the cure-all treatment of further bleeding. Perhaps the unfortunate results of the practice is one reason that moment in history did not last very long. In the twelfth century, bloodletting was practiced by barbers whose red-and-white barber poles became the symbol of their trade.

Historically, phlebotomy used three basic methods. *Venesection* was the most common. A sharp lancet-type instrument pierced the veins and made them bleed. Lancing the veins was thought to eliminate the "bad" blood and remove the disease from the patient. Venesection was often used to reduce fever or to produce a faint so an expectant mother would deliver her baby by the time she recovered.

In *cupping,* a heated glass cup was placed on a person's back. As the cup cooled, it created a suction that pulled blood to the capillaries under the cup. Then a spring-loaded box containing multiple blades cut the area to produce massive bleeding. Both venesection and cupping produced much scarring.

A more modern method was to use *leeches.* It was not uncommon to apply leeches routinely to one's body with the belief it prevented disease. Leeches still have limited uses today. When a person has a reattachment of a finger after accidental amputation, for example, the arteries and veins do not return to normal blood flow immediately. The blood tends to pool in the end of the finger, causing pain and pressure. A leech is placed on the end of the finger to remove the excess blood and relieve the symptoms. The only problem is that the leeches get full rapidly and have to be changed after several hours.

It was not until the middle of the nineteenth century that bloodletting was no longer considered the cure-all for all illnesses. The discovery of microorganisms as the causative agent for many diseases started to change the thinking of how to treat diseases. Blood began to be examined for diagnostic purposes. Urine and feces had been examined since medieval times. The knowledge obtained from these early examinations was small compared with what we can determine today.

Bleeding of individuals to reduce the patient's amount of blood does occur today to treat a disease called polycythemia vera. The treatment involves withdrawing 500 milliliters of blood through therapeutic phlebotomy. But contemporary bloodletting takes a broader approach. Blood is still removed to cure the person, but it is primarily done to find the cure, not as the cure itself. Blood collection has changed from being therapeutic to being diagnostic. There are thousands of different types of diagnostic tests available. Phlebotomy provides accurate and precise test results so the patient can be diagnosed and treated. But this can only be accomplished after the phlebotomist has provided the laboratory with an accurate sample.

PHLEBOTOMY'S ROLE IN HEALTH CARE

The phlebotomist's primary role is to collect blood for accurate and reliable test results as quickly as possible. The job description can vary greatly from one health care environment to another. The phlebotomist is usually cross trained in **venipuncture,** capillary collection, patient care, receptionist duties, and computer work. Phlebotomists have become key players on the health care team. They represent the laboratory and the health care center, they are in direct contact with the patient, and they perform tasks that are critical to the patient's diagnosis and care. Phlebotomists are part of a health care team that can be as large as five thousand people in a large hospital, or two or three in a small clinic.

The traditional role of the phlebotomist in a hospital is only one job: collect patient specimens, primarily blood specimens. A typical day for the traditional phlebotomist is to arrive at work around 0430 and then have a list of patients for collection. Usually this consists of collecting from ten patients on the nursing units and then bringing the specimens to the laboratory at 0530. A second group of patient collection orders is then ready, and the phlebotomist starts on the second round of collections. This consists of fifteen patients who need sample collection no later than 0700. The remainder of the day is spent in returning to the nursing units to collect one or two blood samples at a time as new tests are ordered. Some time is also be spent collecting blood from patients who came in from the outside to have their blood drawn. The evening and night shift phlebotomist waits until a test is ordered to be collected. This single-skilled role for the phlebotomist often results in times of no work and other times of more work than can be done in a short time.

This process works well until there are a large number of patients to draw and the work cannot be completed by 0700. Difficulties in collecting blood from a patient also add a delay to the collection. Getting the blood collected is not the final process. The tests on the blood must be run and the results given to the physician. A physician coming into the hospital to make morning rounds is usually there by 0730, if not sooner, and there would be no results for the physician to review. If the results are not available, the physician must delay treatment of the patient. This results in lengthening of the patient's stay in the hospital.

The problem is in drawing blood from a large number of patients quickly and returning results to the nursing units for the physician to review. The solution is to have more people collecting blood samples during the busy times. It is difficult for a hospital to hire people to come in at 0430 to draw ten patients for an hour and then go home. It is easier to utilize the people who are already working. This includes the current number of phlebotomists and all the nursing staff. Everyone who has contact with the patient needs to become multiskilled. The nurse needs to learn how to collect blood samples, and the phlebotomist needs to learn some of the nursing duties. This has become what is commonly called *patient-focused care.* The duties of the hospital staff revolve more around the patient and the need to treat the patient quickly rather than being restricted to a specific job description. This is similar to the duties of a medical assistant in a physician's office. The job is not restricted to one duty, but multiple tasks are done as the need exists.

The routine in the hospital has become more focused on prompt care of the patient. At 0430 in the morning or sooner, both the nursing staff and the phlebotomist start collecting blood samples. Since more people are collecting the samples, each person does not have as many to collect. As each individual completes sample collection, the samples are sent to the laboratory. This creates a steady stream of specimens flowing to the laboratory. This has eliminated the large batches of work arriving as each phlebotomist finishes. This also means more work is in the laboratory sooner and the laboratory can start working on the testing to get the results available for the physician as morning rounds are made.

When the phlebotomist's blood collection duties are completed, he or she does not return to the laboratory but continues to work on the nursing unit. During the rest of the day, the phlebotomist collects blood samples that are needed, handles patient care, and does laboratory tests such as blood sugars on the patient in the patient's room. This multiskilled training for the phlebotomist makes the phlebotomist more versatile in being an asset to the organization. In some hospitals, this position is known as a *patient care technician.*

Phlebotomists must be familiar with the organization to function in this complex health care field. They usually work directly with the laboratory but indirectly with nurses, physicians, and the staff in the radiology, pharmacy, and physical therapy departments. Many people from different departments need time with the patient. To be better capable of working together, it is best to understand a little about each area.

The phlebotomist often encounters staff from the electrocardiography department. This department does electrocardiograms (abbreviated EKG). An EKG is a recording of impulses of the heart. Impulses from a normal heart make tracing records of a specific size and shape. The abnormal heart shows changes that are different from this pattern. These EKGs are performed in the patient's room, and the phlebotomist often waits for the test to be completed to draw blood.

Another staff member who may visit the patient's room is from the electroencephalography department. This department does electroencephalograms (EEGs), which record the electrical activity of the brain. EEGs help locate and assess the extent of brain injury or determine if there is any brain activity.

The pharmacy department of the hospital is much different from the corner drugstore. The hospital pharmacy dispenses many types of therapeutic drugs that often are much more potent than a prescription taken at home. These drugs are prescribed and monitored under controlled conditions while the patient is in the hospital. The phlebotomist plays an integral part in this monitoring through the blood samples that are collected at specific times. With the results of the samples, the pharmacist is able to consult with the laboratory and the patient's physician. Therapeutic drug monitoring is discussed in more detail in Chapter 6.

The physical therapy department works with patients who due to disease or injury are no longer able to function to their full physical capacity. The therapy may involve rebuilding deteriorated muscles after a long illness or learning to function after an amputation. Related to physical therapy is the department of occupational therapy, where patients work to overcome their physical handicaps so they can be productive again in their old job or function in a new job. Speech therapy is another area related to physical therapy. Patients who have difficulty speaking or who have lost their ability to speak because of a stroke or disease are retaught how to speak.

Radiology is an area of the hospital that has changed rapidly in recent years. Radiologists used to just x-ray lungs or broken bones. But the field has expanded to include cardiac catheterization, CT scans (computed tomography), MRI (magnetic resonance imaging), and ultrasound. Each of these techniques has become a subspecialty of radiology that still looks into the body as the traditional x-ray did, but in a much more detailed and sophisticated way.

The largest department the phlebotomist works with is the department of nursing. Phlebotomists work closely with many of the nurses to give the best care to patients. Phlebotomists may need to ask nurses for assistance with patients who are unwilling to hold still or to check with them about the proper time to draw a specimen. The ability to work with other departments of the hospital is a key trait of the best phlebotomists. The phlebotomist who is well liked and cooperates with others for the patients' care is the one who will earn cooperation from other individuals.

Examples of areas of the hospital are shown in Figure 1.1. The clinical laboratory may be in one location or may be decentralized in a variety of locations in the hospital. These include the main laboratory, ambulatory care laboratory (outpatient laboratory), stat laboratory, or surgery laboratory. Each laboratory serves a specific function and often has sections within it.

Ancillary Hospital Areas and Their Purpose

Administration—Keeps the hospital in compliance

Electrocardiography (EKG)—Monitors cardiovascular patients

Electroencephalography (EEG)—Diagnosis of neurophysiological disorders

Environmental Services—Maintains a clean facility

Food Service (Dietary)—Provides diets to patients

GI Lab—Diagnoses gastrointestinal disorders

Laboratory—Provides testing of patient specimens

Medical Records—Maintains patient records

Nursing—Provides direct patient care

Occupational Therapy—Provides therapy to help maintain living skills

Pharmacy—Dispenses drugs and advises on drug usage

Physical Therapy—Provides therapy to restore mobility

Radiology—Uses imaging for diagnosis and treatment

Respiratory Therapy—Provides therapy to evaluate the lungs

Speech Therapy—Provides therapy to restore speech

Areas of Nursing and Type of Care

Coronary Care Unit (CCU)—Increased care of the patient due to a heart condition

Emergency Department—Emergency treatment of patients

Geriatric—Elderly patients

Home Health Care—Follow-up care of a patient at home

Intensive Care Unit (ICU)—Increased care due the critical needs of the patient

Neonatal—Newborn care

Nephrology—Dialysis patients

Obstetrics—Patient in labor of childbirth

Oncology—Cancer patients

Orthopedic—Patients with broken bones

Pediatrics—Infants and children

Recovery—Recovery treatment of patients

Figure 1.1 *Examples of areas of the hospital.*

The patient-focused care concept takes the laboratory out of a physical location and takes the laboratory to the patient. As instrumentation for laboratory testing becomes smaller, the instrumentation is located on the nursing unit. This testing that is done at the patient's bedside is also known as *point of care testing.* The instrument is taken to the patient's room, the patient's blood is collected, the blood is tested in the instrument, and results are determined at the patient's bedside. This speeds the process of treatment for the patient. A physician can examine the patient, order a blood sugar, and then the patient is tested. Within a few minutes, the physician can have results and decide to continue or change treatment. Bedside testing eliminates the transportation time of the specimen to the laboratory and the wait time to get the results to the nursing unit. However, only a limited number of tests can be performed with the instrumentation available. Federal regulations also limit to some extent what tests can be performed this way. This testing of the blood work at the patient's bedside is often the duty of the multiskilled phlebotomist or nurse.

The laboratory often appears to an outsider like a black box. Into the black box go specimens and out pop the results. This process in turn supports the physician and the hospital, and they in turn support the laboratory. This black box has many sections and functions within it.

The main laboratory is the largest laboratory. The office section of the main laboratory receives and routes laboratory-related telephone calls, specimen collection requests, and some specimens.

In close proximity to the office is the area of specimen collection, more commonly known as phlebotomy. From here the phlebotomists are dispatched to collect blood samples from patients throughout the hospital. The patients are most familiar with this section because often the phlebotomist is the only representative from the laboratory the patient sees. Once collected, the specimens go to any one of the laboratories within the hospital.

The hematology staff studies blood cells and performs qualitative and quantitative analyses along with microscopic examinations. The CBC, or complete blood count (Figure 1.2) is a routine test, providing the physician with a large amount of valuable information about a patients state of health.

Coagulation is usually in the same area as hematology. Coagulation is the study of blood clotting mechanisms. Staff from this section monitor patients on anticoagulant therapy and test patients with bleeding disorders and presurgical patients.

These are groups of tests that have been arranged into panels for general information about a patient's health. These panels are approved for use by the American Medical Association (AMA).

Complete Blood Count (CBC): white blood cell (leukocyte) count and differential white cell count; red blood cell (erythrocyte) count; hematocrit; hemoglobin; red blood cell indices, which include the mean corpuscular volume (MCV), mean corpuscular hemoglobin (MCH), mean corpuscular hemoglobin concentration (MCHC); and the platelet (thrombocyte) count

Electrolyte Panel (Lytes): Sodium, potassium, chloride, CO_2

Hepatic Function Panel: Albumin; total and direct bilirubin; alkaline phosphatase; aspartate aminotransferase (AST), also known as serum glutamic oxaloacetic transaminase (SGOT); alanine aminotransferase (ALT), also known as serum glutamic pyruvic transaminase (SGPT)

Basic Metabolic Panel: Sodium, potassium, chloride, CO_2, glucose, blood urea nitrogen (BUN), and creatinine

Comprehensive Metabolic Panel: Glucose, blood urea nitrogen (BUN), creatinine, sodium, potassium, chloride, calcium, carbon dioxide (CO_2), albumin, total protein, alkaline phosphatase, aspartate aminotransferase (AST), total bilirubin

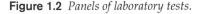

Figure 1.2 *Panels of laboratory tests.*

Staff in the urinalysis section perform qualitative and quantitative chemical and microscopic examinations of urine to detect urinary tract infections, diabetes, and liver or kidney diseases. Urinalysis is often performed in or near the same area as hematology in order to share microscopes.

The chemistry section works with the fluid portion of the blood, the serum or plasma, or other body fluids. The staff perform biochemical analysis of blood and body fluids by manual or automated techniques. A variety of instruments analyze for chemicals such as glucose, electrolytes, blood urea nitrogen (BUN), or creatinine. With almost all instruments, the sample is added to various chemicals, and a color develops. For example, the more the amount of glucose in the blood, the darker the color. In addition to single tests, instruments often run multiple tests on one sample. The panel, a battery of several tests performed on one sample, is a quick, method to screen patients for illness (see Figure 1.2).

Special chemistry is a subsection of chemistry whose staff perform more sophisticated and time-consuming procedures. Examples of these tests are protein electrophoresis, thyroid studies, and aminoglycoside levels.

Microbiology studies organisms that are so small they can only be seen with the aid of a microscope. Here the technologist identifies aerobic and anaerobic bacteria, fungi, mycobacteria (such as tuberculosis), and parasites. Specimens brought to this area include throat cultures, urine cultures, wound and skin cultures, blood cultures, and other types of cultures. Once the organism that is causing the problem is determined, a test called a *sensitivity* is run to determine what antibiotic would be best to eliminate the problem organism.

The immunology section studies antigen–antibody reactions. Antigens are substances seen as being "foreign" in the body, and antibodies are proteins made by the body to combat specific antigens. Staff in this section perform tests to detect and evaluate HIV (human immunodeficiency virus), hepatitis, mononucleosis, rheumatoid arthritis, and syphilis, and they also perform fluorescent antibody tests.

The blood bank section, sometimes called immunohematology, studies antigens and antibodies as they relate to the red blood cells. This section performs blood typing, crossmatching/compatibility testing, and screening for antibodies. The primary testing is to determine compatibility of blood from a donor with a recipient. This crossmatching of donor to recipient determines if the blood that the recipient will receive is **compatible.** Proper patient identification is critical when the blood the phlebotomist draws will be used to determine a product that will be infused into a patient. A misidentification of a patient opens the possibility that the patient will receive the wrong type of blood with serious complications to the patient. The complications can range from fever to death by kidney failure. Few hospitals draw their own donors. Most hospitals procure the blood they transfuse from a central donor facility, such as the Red Cross or local blood centers. Other products that the blood bank issues to patients are platelets and cryoprecipitate.

Cytogenetics is an area found in some of the larger laboratories. This section studies deficiencies that are related to genetic diseases. Genetic testing is expanding rapidly.

The area of cytology and histology, also known as pathology, studies tissues and cell smears to examine them for evidence of cancer, infection, or other abnormalities. All tissue biopsies, surgical specimens obtained in surgery, or tissues obtained in minor surgeries at a physician's office are submitted here for examination. The cytology specimens are processed and then examined microscopically by a cytotechnologist. The majority of the cytology specimens are pap smears. The surgery specimens are prepared by a histologist and then examined macroscopically and microscopically by the pathologist.

The stat laboratory handles stat (emergency) requests. It is staffed twenty-four hours a day, seven days a week. The stat laboratory can do many of the same tests done in the main laboratory, but does these tests individually and not in a batch mode (large groups together), as is often done in the main laboratory. It also provides a backup system for the main laboratory in case of instrument malfunctions.

Near the outpatient entrance of some hospitals, the ambulatory care laboratory (outpatient laboratory) is found. It provides rapid turnaround of results on frequently ordered tests for outpatients. It also has an active marketing and outreach program that includes services for nursing homes, physicians' offices, and health screening for businesses.

Even with the elaborate testing facilities available in most laboratories, outside laboratories are often needed to do specialized testing. These reference laboratories can be in the same city or many miles away. The specimens are transported to the reference laboratory each evening, and results are sent back via computer and telephone lines the next morning.

LABORATORIES IN THE TWENTY-FIRST CENTURY

There is continued pressure on laboratories to produce quality testing in less time for less cost. These pressures are a result of the managed care programs that are in all areas of health care. The emphasis is on increasing outpatient services and decreasing length of stay for inpatients. This puts pressure on the laboratory to do the testing faster and more frequently, so that there is no delay in the physician getting results and being able to treat the patient. The sooner the diagnosis and treatment are determined, the sooner the patient can be on the road to recovery.

Two methods are being used to treat the patient faster with less of a wait on the test results. The first method, mentioned earlier, is point of care testing. The laboratory instrument is taken to the patient, the testing is done in the patient's room, and results are determined at the bedside. The multiskilled phlebotomist often does this type of testing. The results are documented on the patient's chart without any delays. This method of blood testing is usually more expensive than the traditional laboratory test, but often the total cost of care is reduced. With managed care the hospital is often paid one set fee for a patient. The sooner the patient can be released from the hospital, the less it costs the hospital to care for the patient.

Here is an example of how this system works: The managed care provider pays the hospital $1,000.00 per day for a total of five days to care for a patient. It costs the hospital $1,000.00 per day to care for this patient. If the patient takes seven days to be well enough to be released, the costs are $7,000.00, but the hospital will be paid only $5,000.00 by the managed care provider, for a loss of $2,000.00. The incentive for the hospital is to complete the patient's care in less than five days. This is one way the hospital could avoid a loss.

With point of care testing, the test results are available faster. This provides a faster result for the physician to respond to with treatment, and the patient is released sooner. This in turn benefits the patient because the patient is back to a normal lifestyle sooner.

The second method for avoiding a loss is reducing the hospital's cost to below $1,000.00 per day. Consolidation and reengineering of the laboratory are an attempt to make this happen. Laboratories were originally organized around the need to perform inpatient testing. With the emphasis on outpatient surgery and shorter lengths of stay in the hospital, there is an increased demand for outpatient services and presurgery testing. This increase in demand for outpatient services has resulted in hospitals building patient service centers (PSCs) to handle the patients. Patient service centers are located away from the hospital near groups of physician practices. Patients do not have to go all the way to the hospital to get their blood drawn. Patients can have their blood drawn at the service center, which might be in the same building as the physician's office. Patients can even have presurgery work done at the service center and then go to the hospital for surgery. This concept is a benefit to the phlebotomist. Each of these service centers needs to be staffed with a multi-skilled phlebotomist. In the hospital the nursing staff possibly draw the blood, but in the service center the multiskilled phle-botomist collects the samples. The service centers are less expensive to operate than the hospital laboratory. This in turn reduces the costs to the hospital for patient care, resulting in the hospital avoiding a loss in the care of the patient.

Hospitals historically compete for patients. This vigorous competition is evident in newspaper and television advertisement. The laboratory in the hospitals has become a cost that many hospitals wish to remove. Competing hospitals are now forming joint laboratory ventures but still compete vigorously against each other in all other areas. The hospitals join to form a new laboratory company that has each hospital as a part owner and sometimes a commercial reference laboratory as another part owner in this joint venture. The employees of the laboratory become employees of the new company and no longer work for the hospital or commercial laboratory. At the center of this joint venture is what is called a core laboratory. This core laboratory is usually at an off-site location, central to all the hospitals involved. This laboratory is where most of the PSC and outpatient testing are performed. This focuses all the testing from patients not in the hospital to one central core laboratory location instead of multiple hospital locations. The advantage is that only one test instrument must be purchased instead of one instrument for each hospital. This also increases the volume of testing done, and more instrument automation can be implemented to reduce labor costs. With the testing coming in from multiple locations, certain tests that are not very common, called **esoteric** testing, can be performed at the core laboratory. Before the joint venture, no one hospital would have enough volume to do certain tests. By joining forces, certain not so common tests now become common. This provides the physician the ability to order tests and get results back faster than when the testing had to be sent to an out-of-state commercial laboratory.

Hospital laboratories reduce the variety of tests that are completed and concentrate on the tests needed for the immediate care of the inpatient and emergency department patient. These hospital-based laboratories are usually termed rapid response laboratories (RRLs). The key to making all this work is an efficient courier and specimen tracking system. Instead of specimens being walked to another area of the hospital, they have to be transported to another area of the city. To avoid delays, this has to be fast and efficient (see Figure 1.3).

This concept opens up a multitude of opportunities for the phlebotomist. The phlebotomist can do venipuncture in any of the sites or can become multiskilled and rotate to any of the areas, taking on tasks from processing specimens to being a courier. The opportunities become endless for the individual who is willing to learn and rotate to a variety of locations.

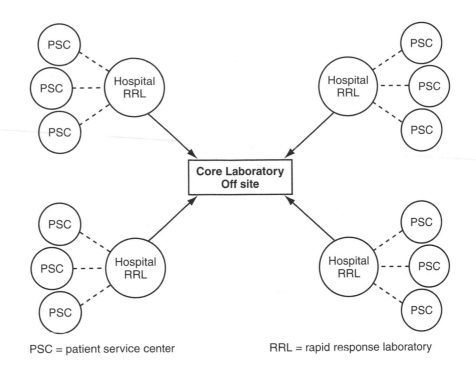

PSC = patient service center   RRL = rapid response laboratory

Figure 1.3 *Core laboratory concept.*

LABORATORY STAFF

The staff working in the laboratory have a large range of duties and training resulting in numerous job titles and roles. The technical positions are either four-year degree positions or two-year associate degree positions. A technologist has a bachelor's degree and a medical technology registry. A technician has a two-year associate degree in medical technology and a registry or certification. Both roles are needed to make a laboratory run smoothly and efficiently. The secretarial or clerical positions in the office areas of the laboratory require a high school education and some secretarial/clerical training. A knowledge of medical terminology is helpful. With advanced medical terminology training and proficient typing ability, the position of medical stenographer could be an option for an advancement.

The phlebotomist position is the one we focus on here. The job of the phlebotomist is to provide specimens for accurate and reliable test results as quickly as possible. The phlebotomist needs a high school education and some specialized training in phlebotomy: a minimum of 40 hours of classroom training and 120 hours of clinical or practical training is the standard set by the American Society of Clinical Pathologists. Individuals with this minimum amount of training may have to work in a clinic, outpatient setting, or small hospital. Once experienced they will be capable of working in a large hospital. Many hospitals and clinics are willing to hire a phlebotomist who has completed only classroom training. The hospital or clinic may offer practical training with the hope that the phlebotomist in training will learn rapidly and be willing to remain at the institution. Many hospitals have established such training programs to fill phlebotomy positions. Phlebotomists may now take certification exams to prove their knowledge in phlebotomy. A variety of certification and registry exams accredit the person as a phlebotomy technician.

Laboratories often employ an individual with a high school education and laboratory experience to work as a laboratory assistant. A laboratory assistant usually has received on-the-job training. A phlebotomist who has shown exceptional abilities and attitude is often considered for such a program. This kind of internship generally occurs in a clinic or small hospital setting. The length of training varies from one health care center to another. After the experience, the laboratory assistant often realizes how enjoyable it is to work in a laboratory and seeks further education to qualify for more demanding job responsibilities and a higher salary. This multiskilling of the phlebotomist opens the opportunities for the phlebotomist to do point of care testing, EKGs, and so on.

The medical laboratory technician, also called a clinical laboratory technician, is a graduate of a two-year associate degree program. This program is taken through a college or proprietary school that is affiliated with a health care center. The health care center provides the practical experience. Once the training is completed, the student must take a certification or registry exam. Some states also have a licensing requirement. Upon successful passing of the certification or registry exam, the technicians are certified as either an MLT (medical laboratory technician) or CLT (clinical laboratory technician).

Another two-year associate degree program that includes at least one year of clinical experience is the histologic technician (HT). The histologic technician prepares the tissue samples for microscopic examination in the histology section of the laboratory. A person who has completed a baccalaureate degree program in histology and a year of histopathology experience will qualify to take the registry exam for histotechnologist.

A section related to histology is cytology. In this section a person with a baccalaureate degree and completion of a twelve-month accredited cytotechnology program is then eligible to take a registry exam to qualify as a CT (cytotechnologist).

Working in the laboratory as a medical technologist requires a baccalaureate degree. This degree involves attending an approved university for three or four years and then spending a full twelve months training in an accredited laboratory. The laboratory portion is equally divided between lectures and working in the laboratory. Once completed, the person may take a registry exam to become an MT (medical technologist). The medical technologist can advance to a supervisor, manager, or administrative director position. The requirements needed to work in a laboratory vary by state.

The person in the laboratory with the most education is the pathologist. The pathologist is a physician who has completed additional schooling and an internship to specialize in **pathology.** This is a physician specialty the same as a pediatrician or a surgeon. The pathologist is sometimes called the doctor's doctor. The physicians within the hospital consult with the pathologist on disease processes they see in a patient. The physicians also confer with the pathologist to determine if additional tests need to be run on a patient to confirm a particular disease process. The pathologist directs the test protocols and test procedures that are done in the laboratory. He or she does extensive consultation on surgical or autopsy specimens, bone marrow procedures, and cytology specimens.

To work in the laboratory, nearly all positions require passing certification and/or state licensing exams. Many agencies certify clinical laboratory personnel. Some of these agencies, the certification, and title they confer are listed here:

Medical Technologist

MT (ASCP): Medical Technologist (American Society of Clinical Pathologists)

MT (AMT): Medical Technologist (American Medical Technologists)

CLT (HHS): Clinical Laboratory Technologist (Department of Health and Human Services)

CLS (NCA): Clinical Laboratory Scientist (National Certification Agency for Medical Laboratory Personnel)

RMT (ISCLT): Registered Medical Technologist (International Society for Clinical Laboratory Technology)

Medical Technician

MLT-AD (ASCP): Medical Laboratory Technician, Associate Degree (American Society of Clinical Pathologists)

MLT-C (ASCP): Medical Laboratory Technician, Certificate (American Society of Clinical Pathologists)

MLT (AMT): Medical Laboratory Technician (American Medical Technologists)

CLT (NCA): Clinical Laboratory Technician (National Certification Agency for Medical Laboratory Personnel)

RLT (ISCLT): Registered Laboratory Technician (International Society for Clinical Laboratory Technology)

Phlebotomist

PBT (ASCP): Phlebotomy Technician (American Society of Clinical Pathologists)

RPT (AMT): Registered Phlebotomy Technician (American Medical Technologists)

CPT (ASPT): Certified Phlebotomy Technician (American Society of Phlebotomy Technicians)

CPT (IAPSI): Certified Phlebotomy Technician (International Academy of Phlebotomy Sciences, Inc.)

CLP (NCA): Clinical Laboratory Phlebotomist (National Certification Agency for Medical Laboratory Personnel)

Phlebotomy Technician (NCCT): (National Center for Competency Testing)

CPT (NPA): Phlebotomy Technician (National Phlebotomy Association)

The agencies and certifications listed are just a few of those available. The phlebotomy area has the most diversification in agencies granting certification. The agency that is accepted worldwide in laboratories for all certification and registries is the American Society of Clinical Pathologists (ASCP). Even though certification has not raised the pay scale for the phlebotomists, it has granted recognition to the phlebotomist as an integral part of the laboratory team.

The laboratory has to be highly organized for the team of laboratory professionals to function smoothly. The interaction can be visualized as an organizational chart for the laboratory that delineates the tasks to be performed, the individuals who are to perform the tasks, and the clinical laboratory as a workplace. Organization defines the relationship among tasks, individuals, and the workplace. The basis for this relationship is authority, responsibility, and accountability. For example, a laboratory manager has the authority attached to the position. If the laboratory manager did not have the position, the manager would not have the authority to hire associates. Responsibility refers to the tasks or duties assigned to the position within the organization. Accountability is the obligation to someone higher on the organizational chart.

An organizational chart is a multilevel vertical hierarchy that signifies the relationship of one position to another. It is sometimes referred to as the chain of command. The larger the organization, the greater the amount of specialization. A laboratory organizational chart develops into a pyramid, with the number of individuals increasing at the base of the pyramid. The laboratory organizational chart usually contains a smaller, adjacent pyramid that includes the pathologists and their relationship to the rest of the laboratory staff. This relationship is shown as a dotted line. Figure 1.4 shows a typical organizational chart.

This organizational chart can be expanded both vertically and horizontally, depending on the size of the laboratory. Communication flows up or down the chart, creating the chain of command. A single laboratory manager is responsible for coordinating the activities for technical procedures, support staff, and achieving goals. Workers receive orders from only one manager or supervisor, and they know who to report to.

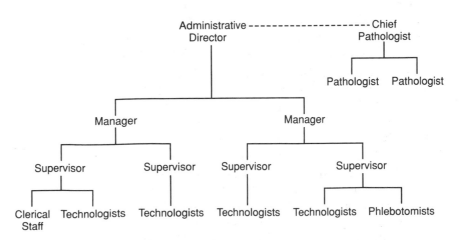

Figure 1.4 *Laboratory organizational chart.*

Phlebotomists play an important role in the health care center. They support the organization and are the main representatives of the quality of the laboratory to the patient. Phlebotomists are professionals and must conduct themselves accordingly. They must maintain a clean and neat appearance and must treat the patient with a gentle touch in a calm and unhurried manner. This role is sometimes difficult to maintain because the patients often do not treat phlebotomists with the respect they deserve.

ETHICAL CONSIDERATIONS

The phlebotomist is intricately involved with ethics and sees ethical decisions being made daily. **Ethics** is hard to define. It consists of more than a set of written rules, procedures, or guidelines. Ingrained in ethics is a moral philosophy that varies by individual, religion, social status, or heritage. Ethics requires that the phlebotomist act responsibly to the patient to provide high-quality patient care. Acting ethically is a standard of conduct a phlebotomist must follow when working with patients and the public. Following this code of ethics is being professional.

Daily patient contact makes the phlebotomist unique among the laboratory associates. Phlebotomists receive training in a manual skill and then are sent to be the laboratory representative throughout the hospital. Phlebotomists have to put up with the worst in human behavior. Patients do not want the phlebotomist to even come near them, and often phlebotomists have to talk and beg the patient into letting them draw the blood. Often patients don't realize that without the work of phlebotomists they would not be able to improve and return home. The nicest patients will often be irritable and may even strike out at the phlebotomist physically when they find themselves in the strange world of the hospital. With this type of abuse, the phlebotomist may find it difficult to be ethical and professional with the patient.

The phlebotomist often has to deal with dying, death, and grief for the first time. Dying is a process. Death is an event. Grief is a response. These can all become very personal when you have worked closely with a patient. Even if the phlebotomist does not experience deep feeling and emotions, the patient and family are very emotional during the process. The emotions generally take five stages:

1. *Denial*—when the family and patient deny reality. ("I will be OK, just let me go home.")

2. *Anger*—when persons express their anger and rage. ("I don't want you to draw my blood. I'm going to die anyway.")

3. *Bargaining*—when persons are willing to do anything to change what has or is happening to them. ("Let me live, I'll change my ways.")

4. *Depression*—when the process is recognized, and there is deep sorrow and feelings over the thought of dying. ("I will do whatever you want to me to do, I don't care.")

5. *Acceptance*—the realistic acknowledgment of the fact they are going to die. ("God's will be done, I am ready.")

The phlebotomist sees the patient at all of these stages. The ability to recognize them helps the phlebotomist to offer sympathy and consoling to the patient and family. The family will often not be on the same stage as the patient. After the patient dies, the family members will usually go through the stages again.

In support of increased ethical treatment of patients and patient relation awareness, the American Hospital Association in 1973 drafted and approved a Patient's Bill of Rights. Their goal was to contribute to more effective care. The Patient's Bill of Rights ensures greater satisfaction of the patient, physician, and hospital. Support of these rights by a hospital should become an integral part of the healing process. This bill of rights existed before the onset of AIDS (acquired immune deficiency syndrome) and before many of the new medical procedures. But it still is very up-to-date in its substance. By following the bill of rights, we are able to see how the patient can be treated ethically and professionally.

Patient's Bill of Rights

The American Hospital Association presents a Patient's Bill of Rights with the expectation that observance of these rights will contribute to more effective patient care and greater satisfaction for the patient, his physician, and the hospital organization. Further, the Association presents these rights in the expectation that they will be supported by the hospital on behalf of its patients, and an integral part of the healing process. It is recognized that a personal relationship between the physician and the patient is essential for the provision of proper medical care. The traditional physician–patient relationship takes on a new dimension when care is rendered within an organizational structure. Legal precedent has established that the institution itself also has a responsibility to the patient. It is in recognition of these factors that these rights are affirmed.

    1. The patient has the right to considerate and respectful care.

    2. The patient has the right to obtain from his physician complete current information concerning his diagnosis, treatment, and prognosis in terms the patient can be reasonably expected to

understand. When it is not medically advisable to give such information to the patient, the information should be made available to
an appropriate person in his behalf. He has the right to know, by
name, the physician responsible for coordinating his care.

3. The patient has the right to receive from his physician information necessary to give informed consent prior to the start of any
procedure and/or treatment. Except in emergencies, such information for informed consent should include but not necessarily be
limited to the specific procedure and/or treatment, the medically
significant risks involved, and the probable duration of incapacita-
tion. Where medically significant alternatives for care or treatment
exist, or when the patient requests information concerning medical
alternatives, the patient has the right to such information. The
patient has the right to know the name of the person responsible for
the procedures and/or treatment.

4. The patient has the right to refuse treatment to the extent
permitted by law and to be informed of the medical consequences
of his actions.

5. The patient has the right to every consideration of his
privacy concerning his own medical care program. Case discussion,
consultation, examination, and treatment are confidential and
should be considered discreetly. Those not directly involved in his
care must have the permission of the patient to be present.

6. The patient has the right to expect that all communications
and records pertaining to his care should be treated as confidential.

7. The patient has the right to expect that within its capacity a
hospital must make reasonable response to the request of a patient
for services. The hospital must provide evaluation, service, and/or
referral as indicated by the urgency of the case. When medically
permissible, a patient may be transferred to another facility only
after he has received complete information and explanation
concerning the needs for and alternatives to such a transfer. The
institution to which the patient is to be transferred must have
accepted the patient for transfer.

8. The patient has the right to obtain information as to any relationship of his hospital to other health care and educational institutions to the extent that his care is concerned. The patient has the
right to obtain information as to the existence of any professional
relationships among individuals, by name, who are treating him.

9. The patient has the right to be advised if the hospital
proposes to engage in or perform human experimentation affecting
his care or treatment. The patient has the right to refuse to participate is such projects.

10. The patient has the right to expect reasonable continuity of
care. He has the right to know in advance what appointment times
and physicians are available and where. The patient has the right to
expect that the hospital will provide a mechanism whereby he is
informed by his physician or a delegate of the physician of the
patient's continuing health care requirements following discharge.

11. The patient has the right to examine and receive an explanation of his bill regardless of source of payment.

12. The patient has the right to know what hospital rules and regulations apply to his conduct as a patient.

No catalog of rights can guarantee for the patient the kind of treatment he has the right to expect. A hospital has many functions to perform, including the prevention and treatment of disease, the education of both health professionals and patients, and the conduct of clinical research. All these activities must be conducted with an overriding concern for the patient, and, above all, the recognition of his dignity as a human being. Success in achieving this recognition assures success in the defense of the rights of the patient.

Most of these rights can be directly applied to duties as a phlebotomist.

1. The patient has the right to considerate and respectful care. Hospitalized patients are out of their normal routine. They may react by being rude or ill-tempered because of their illness or fear. Some patients may be confronting their own mortality for the first time. It is important for the phlebotomist to remain calm and to show consideration and concern for each patient. The phlebotomist also must face the realization of mortality. In the United States, 85 percent of the population dies in the hospital. The phlebotomist will at some time walk into a patient's room and find the patient deceased, possibly before anyone else knows about the death. Even in death the patient must be treated with respect.

2. The physician is the patient's primary source concerning diagnosis and treatment. If questions are asked during the phlebotomy procedure, simply state that the doctor has ordered blood to be drawn for testing, and refer the patient to the physician. The phlebotomist may question the need for the test to be drawn or realize there was an error on a previous specimen, and now the patient has to be redrawn. Questions and concerns should not be discussed with the patient but with the phlebotomist's supervisor or the nurse, outside the presence of the patient.

3. Informed consent. The phlebotomist may need to explain briefly how the venipuncture is performed and that these are tests the doctor has ordered. The patient's act of extending his or her arm for the procedure is taken as an act of consent.

4. Right to refuse treatment. Often by just talking with the patients, they consent to the procedure. If they still refuse, the nursing staff and physician must be informed.

5. Consideration of privacy. It is important to remember to be discreet in approaching the patient. Often the phlebotomist may be in the room at the time another procedure is being performed, the patient is completing personal hygiene, or the physician is examining the patient. Under all of these different circumstances, it is necessary to approach the situation in a mature fashion.

6. Confidentiality. Knowledge concerning a patient's diagnosis is confidential. Matters pertaining to a patient's care should not be discussed in the cafeteria, hallways, or other public areas. Use discretion with such information. Confidentiality can be broken as innocently as finding out that a friend of the family is pregnant and the phlebotomist goes home to tell his or her spouse. The spouse then tells someone else, and all the relatives know before the pregnant woman has had the opportunity to tell anyone.

7. The patient has the right to expect a reasonable response to requests for services. The appropriate person to handle these requests is the nurse and/or physician. Often a patient may request a drink of water, aid in getting out of bed, and so on, from a phlebotomist. Refer these requests to the nursing staff, since the physician may have written specific orders denying the privilege because of upcoming surgery or other aspects related to that patient's care.

8. The patient has the right to know of professional relationships and the names of those who are rendering care. A patient may request the phlebotomist's name and title, and it is appropriate for you to give this information.

9. Experimentation. Patients who are involved in a medical experiment, be it a new drug or treatment, must first be informed of the proposed course of action. The patient must also be informed of its ramifications and must give informed consent to participate in the study.

10. Continuity of care. In these days of multiple specialties and treatment by several physicians at once, it is important to maintain continuity in the care and treatment of patients. For the laboratory this means that specimens should be obtained and processed expeditiously to facilitate the care of the patient.

11. The patient has the right to examine and receive an explanation of his or her bill. Every care should be taken to ensure that the patient is charged for only those tests that are performed and billing is handled expeditiously.

12. The patient has the right to know the hospital rules and regulations that pertain to his or her conduct as a patient.

The application of these rights is not just a perfunctory duty. Part of a caring philosophy is not only to care for the physical and spiritual needs of those in our care, but also to recognize their dignity as human beings. By internalizing this philosophy of caring, not only does the patient benefit; as caregivers we benefit as well.

Central to the job of drawing blood is the patient who is often apprehensive about the procedure we perform. It is important not only to obtain a good specimen, but to do so with a minimal trauma to the patient. Bear in mind that the patient must be treated like anyone would like to be treated. The golden rule is the key to ethical treatment of patients. Proper treatment of the patient and the medical-legal responsibility of the phlebotomist are covered in more detail in Chapters 7 and 8.

The phlebotomist's own attitude toward the job and duties determines how the patient is treated. If the phlebotomist attempts to draw a patient and does not feel confident about obtaining the sample, a "miss" of the patient will probably result. Even when you try to hide it, a negative attitude will resurrect its ugly head and destroy rapport with patients, co-workers, and supervisors. It is not the events of the day that develop the phlebotomist, it is how the phlebotomist deals with those events. The following is a quotation of Charles Swindoll that sums up this impact of attitude and code of ethics for how patients are treated.

Attitude

The longer I live, the more I realize the impact of attitude on life. Attitude, to me, is more important than the past, than education, than money, than circumstances, than failures, than successes, than what any other people think or say or do. It is more important than appearance, giftedness, or skill. It will make or break a company . . . a church . . . a home. The remarkable thing is we have a choice every day regarding the attitude we embrace for that day. We cannot change our past. We cannot change the inevitable. The only thing we can do is play on the one string we have, and that is our attitude. I am convinced that life is 10 percent what happens to me and 90 percent how I react to it. And so it is with you. We are in charge of our attitudes.

A phlebotomist may have ethical questions about continuing care on a terminally ill patient. The phlebotomist must carry out the orders requested by the physician. How extensive the orders and treatment will be depends on the patient and the physician. All states now follow the Patient Self-Determination Act of 1990. This act requires all hospitals participating in Medicare or Medicaid programs to ask all adult inpatients if they have advance directives. The hospital must document the patient's answers and provide information on state laws and hospital policies regarding advance directives.

Formal **advance directives** are documents written before incapacitating illness that state a patient's choices about treatment or name someone to make such choices if the patient becomes unable to make decisions. Through advance directives such as living wills and durable powers of attorney for health care, patients can make legally valid decisions about their future medical treatment.

In a living will a person can stipulate the kind of life-prolonging medical care he or she would want if terminally ill and unable to make medical decisions. In the absence of any advance directive by the patient, the decision is left to the patient's family, physician, and hospital, and sometimes a court of law. Usually the family, physician, and hospital can agree without resorting to the courts, and most states seem to permit this even if it is not clearly stated in the law.

Many hospitals have ethics committees or ethics consultation services, one of whose functions could be to help in decision making about incompetent patients without family or about difficult clinical situations. If the hospital is a religious-based hospital, then its religious affiliation also has an influence on the decisions. Although these ethics committees and religious affiliations often counsel the physician, patient, and family, the final decisions remain the responsibility of the patient, the physician, and the family or other surrogate for the incompetent patient.

STANDARDS USED IN THE LABORATORY

A particular laboratory that serves hospital inpatients is a "hospital laboratory." An "outpatient laboratory" serves only outpatients. The types of patients the laboratory serves determine if that laboratory is governed by a variety of rules and regulations. Abiding by these rules and regulations then determines if that laboratory can qualify for Medicare, Medicaid, and insurance reimbursement. In essence, abiding by these rules and regulations determines whether a laboratory is permitted to function.

There is a large body of regulations governing hospital laboratories and a variety of agencies that issue these regulations and standards. A hospital laboratory accepting Medicare or Medicaid reimbursement must meet all applicable state and local requirements and be accredited by the appropriate agency. It is possible for a hospital to be accredited by the Joint Commission on Accreditation of Healthcare Organizations (JCAHO) or by the American Osteopathic Association (AOA) as a substitute for meeting most of the Medicare requirements. A hospital that has met all the requirements of the JCAHO or AOA will have met almost all the requirements for Medicare. The JCAHO is the accrediting agency most hospitals prefer. The JCAHO was formed in 1951 to give hospitals a way to assure the public of their high standard of care. Since the enactment of the Medicare Act in 1965, the JCAHO has been an acceptable substitute to Medicare accreditation. To prove that the hospital meets standards, the JCAHO sends a team of inspectors to the hospital. The JCAHO now has a three-year accreditation period for hospitals. Once every three years, a team of inspectors visits the hospital to determine if that hospital is still meeting the standards. If the hospital does not pass all of the standards during the inspection, the hospital must correct the deficiencies, prove the correction was made, and/or have a reinspection sooner than three years.

In addition to the hospital meeting the standards of the JCAHO, the laboratory often is inspected voluntarily by another agency, called the College of American Pathologists (CAP). CAP inspects the laboratory and requires it to meet additional standards of performance by sending test samples to the laboratory throughout the year. These test samples must meet the range of results given for that sample on a repeated basis. If the samples continue to fall outside the range, it indicates to the laboratory that the procedure needs to be changed in some way to correct the deficiency. This sample testing gives the laboratory the opportunity to compare itself to other laboratories throughout the country. CAP also sends a team of inspectors to the laboratory to inspect its performance and record keeping. Passing the sample testing requirements and the inspection permits the laboratory to state that it is a CAP-approved laboratory. An added benefit is that JCAHO will often not inspect the laboratory but will accept the CAP inspection as approval enough.

Also checking on the performance of hospitals and laboratories is the individual state board of health. Depending on the particular state, this type of inspection can range from a detailed inspection to just a walk-through of the laboratory. The board of health usually accepts the JCAHO or CAP inspection and then in more detail inspects the rest of the hospital.

To help laboratories maintain the high level of performance necessary to pass these various inspections, the National Committee for Clinical Laboratory Standards (NCCLS), a nonprofit educational organization, was founded in 1968. NCCLS issues publications that describe laboratory procedures, bench and reference methods, and evaluation protocols in all specialties of the laboratory. First, a proposed guideline of procedures is published. Then the users comment on how the guideline can be modified. The NCCLS committee that wrote the document reviews the comments to determine if the guideline should be changed or an appendix should be attached to the document. The document that has gone through the comment period and committee review then becomes a standard. Most of the procedures that are included in the books are based on NCCLS-approved standards. This gives all laboratories approved methods of testing that are consistent nationwide. The publications can be a constant source of reference.

Congress has been involved in the performance standards of the laboratory since it enacted the Clinical Laboratory Improvement Act (CLIA) of 1967. This act mandated comprehensive regulation of laboratories involved in interstate commerce. It was directed at reference laboratories after there was a public outcry about inaccurate testing and kickback payments in the reference laboratory system. As a practical matter, CLIA 1967 does not apply to hospital or physician laboratories. The inspection practices for hospital laboratories just described seem to be sufficient to maintain public and congressional confidence in hospital laboratories' performance. With JCAHO, CAP, and the CLIA 1967, all hospital and reference laboratories had established methods for inspections. The omission was the physician office laboratory that was growing larger and larger as more physicians realized the economic benefits of doing some of their own testing. Laboratories are like all businesses. There are always a few that do not hold rigid standards and turn out substandard results. Some patients were being charged for tests that were not accurate or were even incomplete. Congress then passed a bill called the Clinical Laboratory Improvement Amendments of 1988. These amendments included the physician office laboratories (POLs) in the federal standards and placed quality assurance requirements on other clinical laboratories. CLIA 1988 shifts the focus away from the education and experience qualifications of personnel to the accurate performance of the clinical procedures themselves. This act requires all clinical laboratories to perform quality testing whose accuracy can be proven statistically.

The CLIA 1988 was designed to set safety policies and procedures that protect patients. The standards are based on test complexity and the risk factors associated with incorrect results. The laboratories are monitored by the Health Care Financing Administration (HCFA) of the U.S. Department of Health and Human Services (HHS). They have designated four categories of testing:

1. *Waived tests.* Tests that are simple, unvarying, and require a minimum of judgment and interpretation.

2. *Physician-performed microscopy tests.* Tests the physician personally looks at under the microscope and makes the judgment and interpretation.

3. *Moderate-complexity tests.* Tests that require more complex testing equipment and a moderate amount of judgment and interpretation. Moderate-complexity laboratories must employ personnel with specific levels of education.

4. *High-complexity tests.* Tests that require the most complex testing equipment and a large amount of judgment and interpretation. Highly complex laboratories must employ personnel with specific levels of education.

The moderate-complexity laboratories must have employees who can serve as director, technical consultant, clinical consultant, and testing personnel. The highly complex laboratory has an additional category of general supervisor. These positions do not require successful passing of the certification or registry exams. The position a person can fill is based on his or her educational level and experience (Table 1.1).

Table 1.1	CLIA 1988 PERSONNEL REQUIREMENTS	
CATEGORY	**EDUCATION**	**EXPERIENCE**
1. **Director**	M.D./D.O., pathologist	
	M.D./D.O.	1 year of experience
	Ph.D.	
	M.S.	2 years' experience or training
	B.S.	4 years' experience or training
2. **Technical Consultant**	M.D./D.O., pathologist	
	M.D./D.O.	1 year of experience
	Ph.D. or M.S.	1 year of experience or training
	B.S.	2 years' experience or training
3. **Clinical Consultant**	M.D./D.O., pathologist	
	M.D./D.O.	1 year of experience
	Ph.D.	Board certified
	M.D./D.O.	State licensed
4. **Testing Personnel**	M.D./D.O.	
	Ph.D., M.S.	
	B.S.	In appropriate science
	Associate degree	In appropriate science
	High school diploma	Appropriate training
5. **General Supervisor**	Director	
	M.D./D.O.	
	Ph.D., M.S. or B.S.	1 year of experience
	Associate degree	2 years' experience

To qualify for a category, the employee must meet one or more of the education and experience requirements.

The goal of the regulations just discussed is to protect the patient. These regulations work to assure that accurate and reliable testing methods are being used to provide the best results to the patient. The Occupational Safety and Health Act (OSHA) of 1970 regulates the safety and protection of the associate doing testing. *The Federal Register Rules and Regulations* of December 6, 1991, established new regulations that employers must follow to protect their associates from blood or other potentially infectious materials. The enforcement of the act started on July 6, 1992. This act dictates that the employer is responsible for enforcing the rules and OSHA can issue fines of up to $7,000 per infraction. The range of this act is far reaching and affects all associates and patients of the health care system. The implementation of these regulations can have a financial impact, but their purpose is to provide a safe work environment. Chapter 2 presents more details of the OSHA rules and regulations.

QUALITY ASSURANCE IN PHLEBOTOMY

Phlebotomists must realize that quality is their responsibility. The result of the test that is sent to the physician depends on the quality of the sample that the phlebotomist obtains. A sample drawn from the wrong patient or a sample that is contaminated or clotted will give inaccurate results. A variety of agencies work to ensure that health care facilities meet standards, rules, and regulations. To monitor the compliance to these standards, rules, and regulations, several programs within the health care facility are utilized. One such program is a quality assurance program. This program strives to have the health care facility guarantee that all areas are providing the highest quality and most appropriate patient care. The quality assurance program must contain an element of quality control for the program to function. Quality control comprises the methods of monitoring the processes that are providing patient care: that is, equipment maintenance and calibration of equipment, following phlebotomy standards.

The JCAHO has outlined ten steps to a quality assurance plan:

1. Assign responsibility.
2. Delineate scope of care.
3. Identify important aspects of care.
4. Identify indicators related to these aspects of care.
5. Establish thresholds for evaluation.

6. Gather and organize data.

7. Evaluate care when thresholds are reached.

8. Take corrective action.

9. Assess the effectiveness of the actions; document improvement.

10. Communicate relevant information.

To supplement this plan, the health care facility must also have a total quality management (TQM) and continuous quality improvement (CQI) plan in place. The TQM plan is a management plan that ensures that the quality expected can be met. This plan establishes the ensurance of adequate supplies and personnel, up-to-date procedures, and acceptable patient outcomes (the patient's health improving). The CQI plan aims at more than just meeting the minimum standards. The CQI plan does not accept the status quo; there must be constant efforts to improve what is being done. Both plans focus on the entire health care team seeking customer satisfaction as the final outcome. The phlebotomist must monitor a variety of quality improvement items. Seven examples follow:

1. Phlebotomist response time (for inpatients)

2. Patient waiting (for outpatients)

3. Time it takes to do a phlebotomy procedure

4. Number of redraws due to inappropriate amount of specimen

5. Number of incorrect tubes drawn

6. Number of patients requiring a second attempt

7. Number and size of hematomas

BODY SYSTEMS

The human body has a variety of body systems and functions. Homeostasis and metabolism are two of the main body functions. The body maintains its own internal environment of many processes that work both independently and together to maintain an equilibrium. When all parts work together to maintain a steady state, the body is maintaining homeostasis. Consider a person with anemia. In anemia, the person does not have enough hemoglobin, or red blood cells, to provide oxygen in adequate amounts to all parts of the body. The entire body slows down, and the person has little energy, so not as much oxygen is needed.

Metabolism in the body is the process of making substances or breaking down substances so the body can function. Catabolism is the process of producing energy by breaking down complex compounds into simple ones. This is the way that energy is provided to all parts of the body. Anabolism is the constructive part of metabolism in which the body uses simple substances to build substances. The body is constantly replacing itself to maintain a healthy individual. Skin grows over a cut to heal the injury. Blood cells are constantly being created, demonstrating the need for anabolism. Through these body functions, nonliving material is converted into the living cytoplasm of the cell.

Skeletal System

The skeletal system of the body supports movement. There are over two hundred bones in the human body that provide this support. The bone marrow within many bones of the skeletal system provides much of the blood for the circulatory system. The health of the skeletal system can be analyzed by checking the patient's analytes, such as calcium and phosphate levels and the synovial fluid.

Muscular System

The musculoskeletal system is responsible for both internal and external movement. The heart is a muscle that helps move the blood through the circulatory system. Contraction and relaxation of muscles attached to bones provide movement. The muscular system is analyzed by direct muscle biopsy or muscle enzyme testing.

Nervous System

The nervous system provides the communication lines for the different systems and knows what each system needs. Testing of the cerebral spinal fluid is one way the laboratory checks the function of this system.

Respiratory System

The respiratory system maintains the body's ability to exchange gases. The lungs take in oxygen and transfer it to the red blood cells. At the same time the lungs expel the carbon dioxide that the red blood cells have brought back from all parts of the body. This circulation of the blood and exchange of gases provides the much needed oxygen to the tissue cells. The testing of the respiratory system is done by drawing arterial blood gases.

Urinary System

The urinary system's primary function is to eliminate fluids and wastes through urine. The kidneys are the main part of this system and work to regulate the amount of water and solutes the body system expels. A variety of urine and blood tests such as BUN or creatinine analyze the function of the urinary system.

Digestive System

The digestive system helps the body system to absorb food that the tissue cells need. The body system then uses this absorbed food in metabolism to generate energy or build substances. This system eliminates the wastes from the body.

Endocrine System

The endocrine system is composed of glands that manufacture and secrete substances needed by the body. There are two kinds of glands in this system: exocrine and endocrine. The exocrine glands discharge through ducts or tubes either into the intestines or outside of the body. They consist of tear glands, sweat glands, salivary glands, mucous glands, and mammary glands, to name a few. Endocrine glands release their products directly into the bloodstream. Some of the endocrine glands are the pituitary glands, thyroid glands, parathyroid glands, and adrenal glands. They are often called ductless or internal glands. The substances produced are hormones. The hormones have a powerful effect on the body by controlling growth, the shape of the body, and the way the body reacts to fright or anger. Each of these glands must maintain a balance to allow the body to adjust to the outside world and maintain health.

Reproductive System

The reproductive system consists of a male system and a female system. The male system's main function is to produce sperm and hormones. The most important male hormone is testosterone. The female system's main function is to produce eggs and hormones. The most predominant female hormones are estrogen and progesterone.

Circulatory System

Each body system works together simultaneously to provide other body systems the necessary products or energy they need. The circulatory system is the way the body transfers substances and wastes from one system to another. The circulatory system is the system of the body that the phlebotomist should be most knowledgeable about, and we discuss it in detail in the next section.

The lymphatic system is considered part of the circulatory system. This system circulates lymph fluids to parts of the body and also produces blood cells. It is also discussed in more detail in the next section.

ANATOMY AND PHYSIOLOGY OF THE CIRCULATORY SYSTEM

To be prepared to collect blood, you must understand the system that carries this blood: the circulatory system. The bone marrow is the primary factory for production of blood cells. The lymph nodes, thymus, and spleen are also sites for the production of blood cells. The function of blood is to carry oxygen to body tissues and to remove the waste product carbon dioxide. The blood also carries nutrients to all parts of the body and moves the products to the lungs, kidneys, liver, and skin.

The body contains approximately 5 liters of blood. Forty-five percent consists of formed elements, and 55 percent is a fluid portion, called plasma. Generally 2.0 milliliters of blood yields about 1 milliliter of fluid. The formed cellular elements consist of **erythrocytes** (red blood cells), **leukocytes** (white blood cells), and **thrombocytes** (platelets) (see Figure 1.5 and Table 1.2).

The blood cells begin their formation in the bone marrow and lymph nodes as undifferentiated **hemopoietic** stem cells. Through **hemopoiesis** they continue to mature through different stages, slowly decreasing in size. When the cells leave the bone marrow and enter the bloodstream, they consist of mature cells. If immature cells are found in the bloodstream, this is indicative of a hematological problem (see Figure 1.6).

Mature erythrocytes average 7–8 micrometers in diameter and are biconcave in shape, living about 120 days once they enter the bloodstream. Mature erythrocytes have no nucleus. The cells consist of a membrane that encases hemoglobin. Hemoglobin is the iron-containing pigment of the red blood cells. The hemoglobin holds oxygen molecules that were absorbed through the membrane as the erythrocytes passed

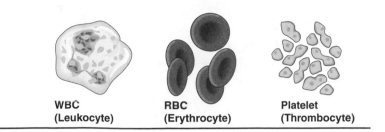

WBC
(Leukocyte)   RBC
(Erythrocyte)   Platelet
(Thrombocyte)

Figure 1.5 *Formed cellular elements of the blood. Note. From* Comprehensive Medical Assisting, Administrative and Clinical Competencies *(p. 823), by W. Lindh, M. S. Pooler, D. C. Tamparo, and J. U. Cerrato, 1998, Albany, NY: Delmar Publishers. Copyright 1998 by Delmar Publishers. Reprinted with permission.*

Table 1.2	CELLULAR ELEMENTS OF THE BLOOD		
	WBC *(Leukocyte)*	**RBC** *(Erythrocyte)*	**PLATELET** *(Thrombocyte)*
Function	Body defense	Transport of oxygen and carbon dioxide (intravascular)	Stoppage of bleeding
Formation	Bone marrow, lymphatic tissue	Bone marrow	Bone marrow
Size/shape	9–16 micrometers; different size, shape, color nucleus (core)	6–7 micrometers biconcave disc. Normally no nucleus in mature cells found in bloodstream	1–4 micrometers; fragments of megakaryocytes
Life span	Varies, 24 hours–years	100–120 days	9–12 days
Normal values	3,500–11,000/ cubic millimeter	3.8–5.9 million/ cubic millimeter	150,000–400,000/ cubic millimeter
Removal	Bone marrow, liver, spleen	Bone marrow, liver, spleen	Spleen

through the lungs. The hemoglobin then releases the oxygen to tissues and brings carbon dioxide back to the lungs to be released as a waste product. An anemic person has too little hemoglobin. Many anemic individuals also have a decreased number of erythrocytes.

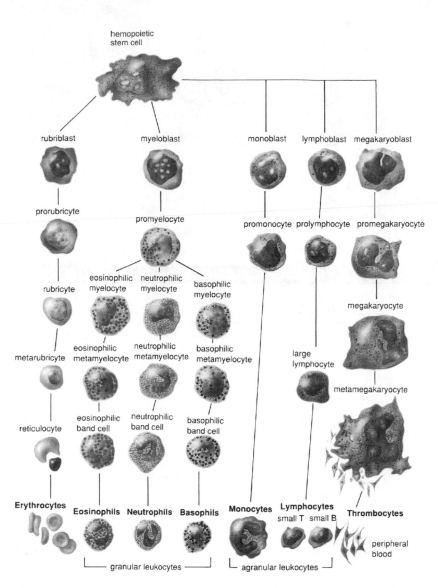

Figure 1.6 *Hemopoiesis showing blood cells and platelet formation starting with hemopoietic stem cell. Note. From* Comprehensive Medical Assisting, Administrative and Clinical Competencies *(p. 848), by W. Lindh, M. S. Pooler, D. C. Tamparo, and J. U. Cerrato, 1998, Albany, NY: Delmar Publishers. Copyright 1998 by Delmar Publishers. Reprinted with permission.*

The membrane of the erythrocyte does more than just encase the hemoglobin. The erythrocytes contain antigens on the surface that determine the individual's blood type and a variety of other factors specific for that individual. Antibodies that can react with antigens foreign to the individual are found in the patient's plasma. These antigen–antibody reactions are important when blood is transfused into an individual. The process of determining if a person will react after a transfusion is called a type and cross-match (T&C). The blood bank section of the laboratory performs the T&C. It is of a critical importance that the phlebotomist drawing a blood sample be absolutely positive about patient iden-tification. From the sample the phlebotomist draws, the blood bank determines what blood to give the patient.

The bone marrow and lymph nodes produce the leukocytes. The leukocytes start as undifferentiated stem cells just like the erythrocytes and then form into blast cells, maturing through several stages until they are released into the blood as mature cells (Figure 1.6).

The leukocytes vary greatly in size. They appear as large white cells that have purple centers (nuclei) when viewed in a blood smear. Some of the cells also have granules that stain pink, blue, or orange. These staining characteristics help to identify the different cells. When a technologist counts at least a hundred of these leukocytes and classifies them according to the percentage of cell types that are found, the physician receives a report called a white blood cell differential count. This differential count changes depending on the disease process that is taking place. A differen-tial count can indicate whether a person has a viral infection, bacterial infection, appendicitis, and so on. Figure 1.7 illustrates the six basic types of mature leukocytes and their comparative sizes.

This differential count is only part of a complete blood count (CBC). The rest of the CBC contains the number of white blood cells, red blood cells (RBCs), hemoglobin, and hematocrit of the patient. Calculations involving the hemoglobin, hematocrit, and RBCs give the physician facts called the indices of the RBC. All of this information can give the physician a general screening of the patient's health. Figure 1.8 shows a CBC report form.

The thrombocytes (platelets) are the smallest of the formed elements. They are fragments of cells that break off from a large cell called a metamegakaryocyte, found in the bone marrow. The function of the thrombocytes is to aid in the clotting process. When a person is cut, the platelets are the first cells to go to the

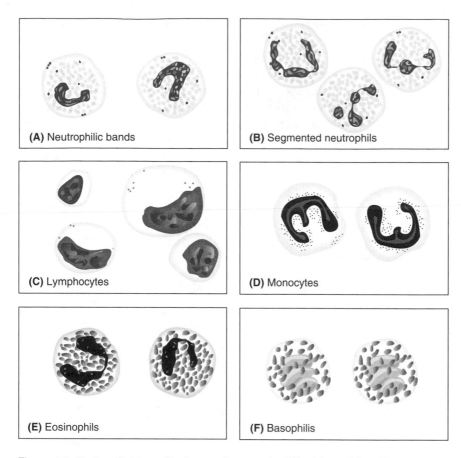

Figure 1.7 *Various divisions of leukocytes from a stained blood smear. Note. From* Comprehensive Medical Assisting, Administrative and Clinical Competencies *(p. 869), by W. Lindh, M. S. Pooler, D. C. Tamparo, and J. U. Cerrato, 1998, Albany, NY: Delmar Publishers. Copyright 1998 by Delmar Publishers. Reprinted with permission.*

site. They start sticking together to try to plug the hole. Then other clotting factors become active to complete the clotting process. The thrombocyte matures from an undifferentiated stem cell just like the erythrocytes and leukocytes (Figure 1.6).

The heart pumps the blood through the body by way of tubing called arteries, veins, and capillaries. When blood flows away from the heart, it flows in the artery. Blood flowing back to the heart flows in the veins. Connecting most of the arteries and veins are the capillaries (Figure 1.9).

The artery has a thick wall that helps it withstand the pressure of the pumping of the heart. We can use the analogy of the body

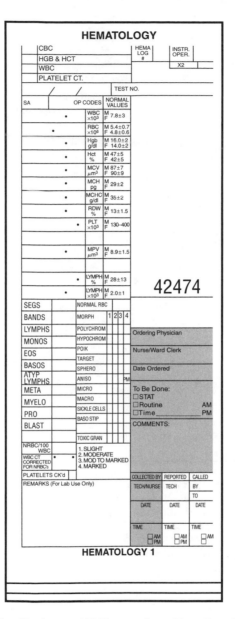

Figure 1.8 *Complete blood count (CBC) report form. Note. From* Comprehensive Medical Assisting, Administrative and Clinical Competencies *(p. 849), by W. Lindh, M. S. Pooler, D. C. Tamparo, and J. U. Cerrato, 1998, Albany, NY: Delmar Publishers. Copyright 1998 by Delmar Publishers. Reprinted with permission.*

ARTERIES VERSUS VEINS	
Arteries	**Veins**
1. Carry blood from the heart, carry oxygenated blood (except pulmonary artery)	1. Carry blood to the heart, carry deoxygenated blood (except pulmonary vein)
2. Normally bright red in color	2. Normally dark red in color
3. Elastic walls that expand with surge of blood	3. Thin walls/less elastic
4. No valves	4. Valves
5. Can feel a pulse	5. No pulse

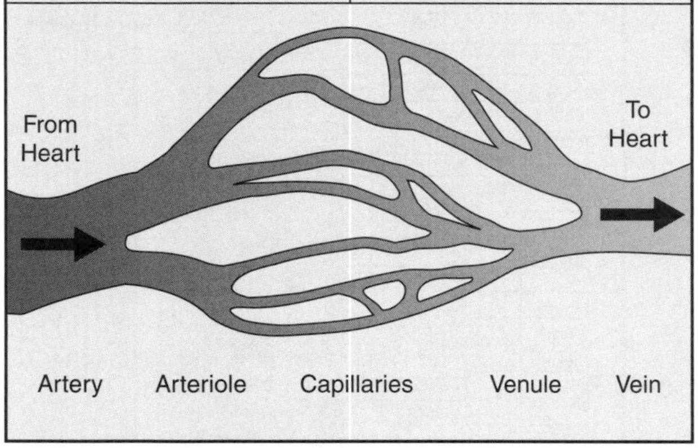

From Heart → Artery   Arteriole   Capillaries   Venule   Vein → To Heart

Figure 1.9 *Blood flow: Oxygenated blood in the arteries becomes deoxygenated upon leaving the capillaries and entering the veins. Note. From* Comprehensive Medical Assisting, Administrative and Clinical Competencies *(p. 822), by W. Lindh, M. S. Pooler, D. C. Tamparo, and J. U. Cerrato, 1998, Albany, NY: Delmar Publishers. Copyright 1998 by Delmar Publishers. Reprinted with permission.*

builder who has built his muscles to the point of being stronger and thicker. The arteries are constantly expanding and contracting and therefore have a thicker, stronger wall. The arteries start branching off to form arterioles that branch even more to become capillaries. The capillaries then start forming together to form venules, and the venules then become veins. As blood flows through the body, it follows this path of artery–capillary–vein. Oxygenated arterial blood leaves the heart and carries this oxygen to the tissue by releasing the oxygen through the cell walls of the capillaries. At the same time, carbon dioxide is being absorbed by

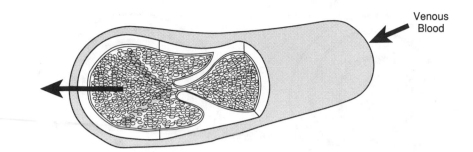

Venous
Blood

Figure 1.10 *Valve.*

the blood and then transported to the lungs to be exhaled as a
waste product. The flow of the blood also regulates body temperature. When the body gets warm, the capillaries in the extremities
dilate (enlarge in diameter) and let off heat. This process then
cools the body. If the body becomes cold, the capillaries constrict
(get smaller in diameter) and less blood flows through, therefore
conserving heat for the rest of the body. That is why our feet and
fingers get cold before other parts. When we discuss microcollection in Chapter 5, we see that heat stimulation of blood flow is
very useful.

To keep the blood flowing in a one-way direction, the veins in
the extremities contain structures called valves. These valves let
the blood pass through but close shut if the blood tries to flow
backward (Figure 1.10).

If you look more closely at the structure of the arteries and
veins, you can see they are not made of one monolayer of tubing
but have multiple layers. The cells in these layers run in
different directions and give strength to the arteries and veins
(Figure 1.11). It is like a piece of plywood. Plywood is stronger
than a piece of wood the same thickness because the lamination
of the plywood has given it strength. This layering also helps
keep the arteries and veins from rupturing and splitting when
punctured with a needle to draw blood.

As was already explained, the formed elements of the blood
make up only 45 percent of the total volume. The remaining
55 percent is liquid. In the body, the liquid portion is called
plasma. When the blood is removed from the body, the blood clots
and the liquid portion are called **serum.** The clot contains all the
formed elements intertwined together in a fibrin mass. Blood that
is flowing through the body contains a protein called fibrinogen.
Once the blood leaves the body, the fibrinogen turns into fibrin.

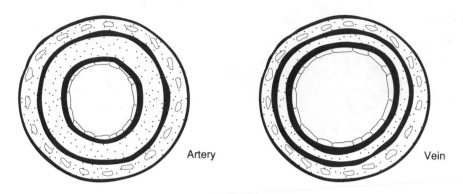

Figure 1.11 *Wall structure.*

1. Uncoagulated blood
2. Calcium utilized
3. Prothrombin converts to thrombin
4. Fibrinogen converts to fibrin
5. Clot formation with serum extracted

Figure 1.12 *Steps to a clot.*

This fibrin is like a sticky spider web and traps the formed
elements into the fibrin mass called a clot. The clot then contracts,
and the liquid (serum) portion is extracted (Figure 1.12). This
serum is a clear straw-colored liquid that is used for many of the
tests done in the laboratory. To speed the removal of the serum, an
instrument called a **centrifuge** spins the blood. A carrier holds the
tubes of blood in an upright position, and when the centrifuge is
started, the carriers spin in a circle. This is similar to a weight on
the end of a string. The string is vertical, but as the weight is
swung in a circle, the weight assumes a horizontal position. The
carriers in the centrifuge must be balanced and assume a horizontal position to push the blood to the bottom of the tube, much
like what happens in a washing machine as the clothes are pushed
to the outside of the washer (Figure 1.13). The blood separates
according to weight. The clot then goes to the bottom of the tube,
and the serum is on the top layer. This separation of the blood is
due to the centrifical force on the blood.

To produce a plasma specimen, the blood has to be
prevented from clotting. An **anticoagulant** is a chemical

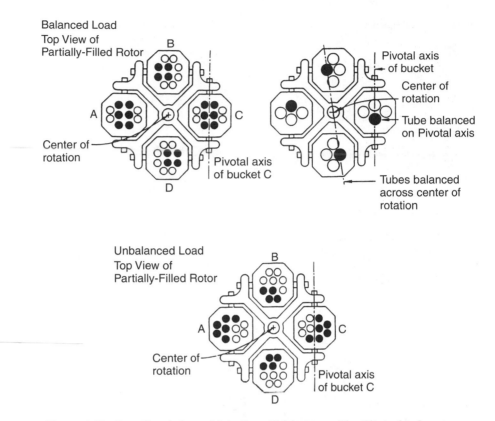

Figure 1.13 *Centrifuge balance. Note. From* Phlebotomy: The Clinical Laboratory Manual Series *(p. 13), by L. Hoeltke, 1995, Albany, NY: Delmar Publishers. Copyright 1995 by Delmar Publishers. Reprinted with permission.*

substance that prevents the blood from clotting by preventing the fibrinogen from converting to fibrin. Putting a small amount of anticoagulant into a test tube prevents the blood from clotting and keeps it in a condition similar to how it was in the body. An anticoagulated tube of blood that has been centrifuged layers the formed elements and plasma according to weight. The bottom layer contains the erythrocytes, and there is a thin layer called the **buffy coat.** The buffy coat contains a mixture of leukocytes and thrombocytes. On top of all these layers is the plasma layer. The plasma contains fibrinogen and usually is slightly hazy (Figure 1.14).

The heart, the organ that keeps all of this blood flowing, is a muscle with four distinct chambers: the right atrium, right ventricle, left atrium, and left ventricle (Figure 1.15). Blood enters the heart through the right atrium and left atrium. Blood leaves the heart by way of the right and left ventricles. The right side of the heart is

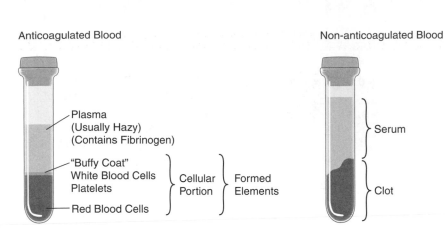

Anticoagulated Blood

Plasma
(Usually Hazy)
(Contains Fibrinogen)

"Buffy Coat"
White Blood Cells
Platelets

Red Blood Cells

Cellular
Portion

Formed
Elements

Non-anticoagulated Blood

Serum

Clot

Figure 1.14 *Blood tubes. Note. From* Comprehensive Medical Assisting, Administrative and Clinical Competencies *(p. 824), by W. Lindh, M. S. Pooler, D. C. Tamparo, and J. U. Cerrato, 1998, Albany, NY: Delmar Publishers. Copyright 1998 by Delmar Publishers. Reprinted with permission.*

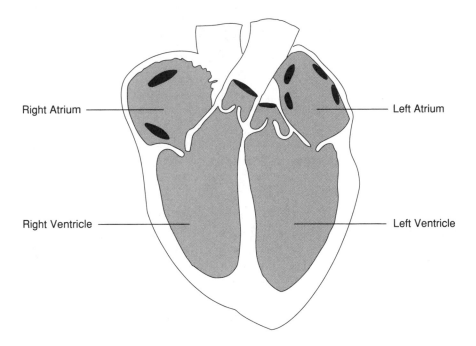

Right Atrium

Left Atrium

Right Ventricle

Left Ventricle

Figure 1.15 *Heart chambers.*

responsible for oxygenating the blood by pumping it to the lungs. The left side of the heart has the task of pumping the blood to all parts of the body. The blood flows through the body via the arteries, arterioles, capillaries, venules, and veins (Table 1.3). A muscular wall called the septum divides the right and left sides of the heart.

Table 1.3   BLOOD FLOW CHART

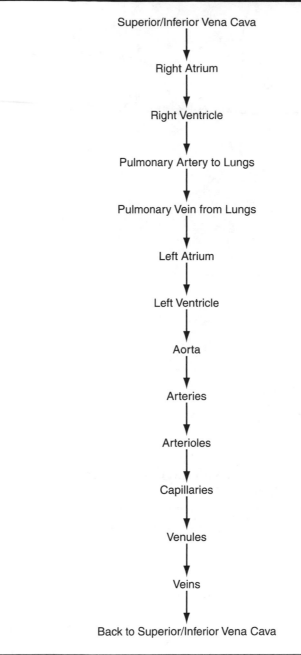

Superior/Inferior Vena Cava

↓

Right Atrium

↓

Right Ventricle

↓

Pulmonary Artery to Lungs

↓

Pulmonary Vein from Lungs

↓

Left Atrium

↓

Left Ventricle

↓

Aorta

↓

Arteries

↓

Arterioles

↓

Capillaries

↓

Venules

↓

Veins

↓

Back to Superior/Inferior Vena Cava

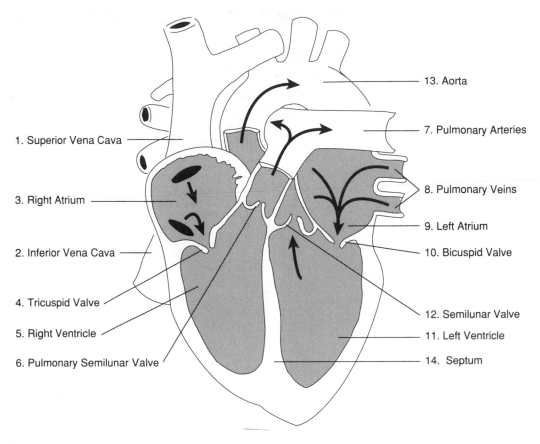

1. Superior Vena Cava

3. Right Atrium

2. Inferior Vena Cava

4. Tricuspid Valve

5. Right Ventricle

6. Pulmonary Semilunar Valve

13. Aorta

7. Pulmonary Arteries

8. Pulmonary Veins

9. Left Atrium

10. Bicuspid Valve

12. Semilunar Valve

11. Left Ventricle

14. Septum

Figure 1.16 *Heart.*

Referring to Figure 1.16, you can follow the flow of blood through the heart. Blood that has given up its oxygen (deoxygenated blood) enters the heart from the upper part of the body by way of the *superior vena cava*. Blood from the lower part of the body enters the heart by way of the *inferior vena cava*. The first chamber of the heart this deoxygenated blood enters is the *right atrium*. The blood then passes through the *tricuspid valve* and enters the *right ventricle*. The tricuspid valve is a one-way valve that keeps the blood from flowing back into the right atrium. From the right ventricle the deoxygenated blood passes through the *pulmonary semilunar valve* (pulmonary valve) into the *pulmonary artery*. The pulmonary artery leaves the heart and enters the lungs. The pulmonary artery branches in the lungs into millions of capillaries. In the lungs, the blood releases the carbon dioxide it picked up while passing through the body and becomes oxygenated. The pulmonary artery is the only artery in the body that carries deoxygenated blood.

Once the blood leaves the lungs it enters the *pulmonary veins* for its trip back to the heart. The pulmonary vein is the only vein in the body that carries oxygenated blood. The blood now has a bright red appearance because of the oxygen it is holding. The pulmonary veins enter the heart at the left atrium. The oxygenated blood of the left atrium flows through the *bicuspid valve* (also known as mitral valve) into the *left ventricle*. The left ventricle pumps the blood through another valve called the *semilunar valve* (also known as aortic valve). From here the blood enters the largest artery in the body, the *aorta*. The aorta branches to become the entire artery system of the body. To pump this blood to all parts of the body, the left ventricle produces extreme pressure. This one last pump has to be sufficient to pump the blood all the way to the tip of the toes and back to the heart. This is why the left ventricle has such a thick wall. This chamber of the heart has built up its muscles to be thicker and stronger.

A sac called the pericardium encloses the heart. The heart itself has three layers of tissue. The *endocardium* is a membrane layer that lines the inner chambers of the heart and the valves. The *myocardium* is the muscle of the heart itself. The *epicardium* is the outermost membrane layer of the heart. **Endocarditis** is an infection of the endocardium of the heart. If untreated, the endocarditis can destroy the heart valves by eating away part of the tissue. This causes the valves to fail to open or close properly. In severe cases the valve may need to be replaced in open heart surgery.

The heart pumps oxygenated blood to all parts of the body. While the blood is in the heart, it does not supply oxygen to the heart. Coronary arteries supply this oxygen to the surface of the heart. Coronary veins on the surface of the heart remove the carbon dioxide (Figure 1.17). The arteries branch off the aorta and supply the heart with the oxygen it needs to survive. If one or more of these coronary arteries become **occluded,** the myocardium in that area of the heart dies and a myocardial infarct (heart attack) is the result. Numerous surgical techniques can correct these occlusions if caught soon enough.

The chambers of the heart do not pump independently with each chamber pumping at a different time. The heart is a double pump with both sides of the heart pumping almost simultaneously. Both ventricles expand at the same time while the atria are contracting, pulling blood from the right and left atrium. The appropriate valves close, and the ventricles then contract to push the blood to the lungs and through the aorta at the same time.

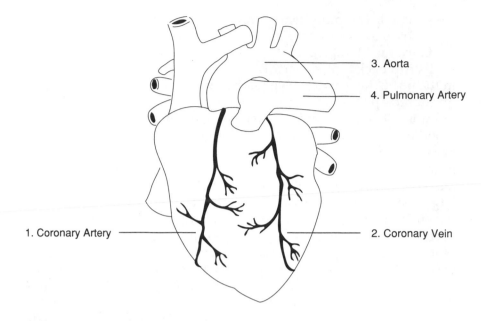

Figure 1.17 *Coronary arteries and veins.*

Electrical stimuli control the pumping action of the heart. The specialized cardiac tissue controlling the electrical stimuli is the conduction system of the heart (Figure 1.18). The sinoatrial node (SA node) begins the process. The SA node needs no outside stimulus to cause it to start a heartbeat. Therefore the SA node is known as the pacemaker of the heart. The SA node creates an electrical impulse that is transmitted to the atrioventricular node (AV node). The AV node then causes the atria to contract. The electrical impulse then travels a length of conduction fibers called the bundle of His to the right and left ventricle. The right and left ventricle have fibers called Purkinje's fibers running up and down the ventricles. These Purkinje's fibers cause the ventricles to contract. If this electrical pathway starts to fail, it may be corrected by a cardiac pacemaker.

As the heart pumps it creates a pressure in the arteries of the body. The **systolic** pressure is the pressure when the heart is contracted. The **diastolic** pressure is the pressure when the heart is relaxed between beats. Blood pressure is read as 120/80: the 120 is the systolic pressure, and the 80 is the diastolic pressure. The pressures are recorded as 120 mm Hg. The mm Hg refers to millimeters of mercury.

The antecubital fossa (bend of the arm) is the usual location where the phlebotomist chooses to draw blood. The veins are near the surface and large enough to give access to the blood

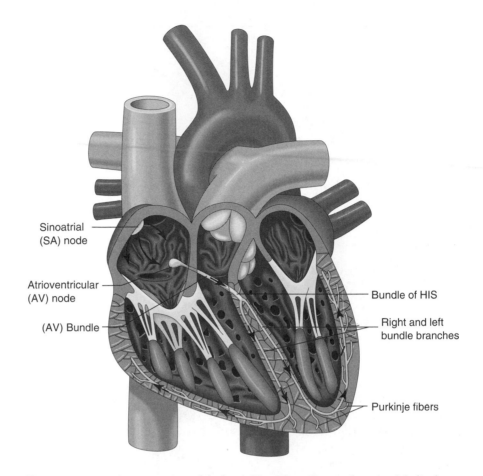

Sinoatrial
(SA) node

Atrioventricular
(AV) node

(AV) Bundle

Bundle of HIS

Right and left
bundle branches

Purkinje fibers

Figure 1.18 *Conduction system of the heart. Note. From* Comprehensive Medical
Assisting, Administrative and Clinical Competencies *(p. 764), by W. Lindh, M. S.
Pooler, D. C. Tamparo, and J. U. Cerrato, 1998, Albany, NY: Delmar Publishers.
Copyright 1998 by Delmar Publishers. Reprinted with permission.*

(Figure 1.19). The median cubital vein is the vein that is used the
majority of the time. When this vein is not available, any of the
other veins that can be felt may be used. These veins include the
basilic, cephalic, median, and median cubital. The superficial
veins in the hand require special techniques for collection.

The arteries in the arm consist of the brachial artery in the
brachial region of the arm and the radial and ulnar arteries in the
wrist (Figure 1.20). Puncturing of arteries requires special techniques, used when obtaining a blood gas specimen. Arterial
punctures and the techniques used to draw blood from these
locations for blood gas testing are explained in Chapter 4.

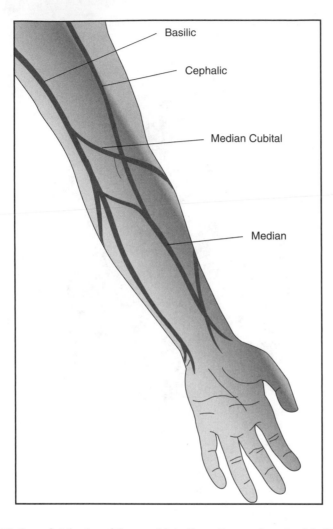

Basilic

Cephalic

Median Cubital

Median

Figure 1.19 *Superficial veins of the arm. Note. From* Comprehensive Medical Assisting, Administrative and Clinical Competencies *(p. 824), by W. Lindh, M. S. Pooler, D. C. Tamparo, and J. U. Cerrato, 1998, Albany, NY: Delmar Publishers. Copyright 1998 by Delmar Publishers. Reprinted with permission.*

The veins of the feet are an alternative when the arms are not available. A physician's permission is needed before drawing blood from the veins of the legs and feet (Figure 1.21). The physician may not want the patient's leg or foot veins punctured, because the act of drawing blood may cause clots to form. These clots could dislodge and cause a blockage elsewhere in the body.

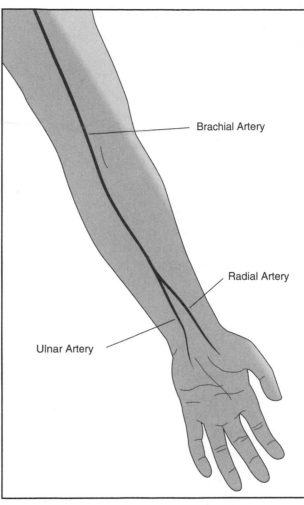

Figure 1.20 *Arteries of the arm. Note. From* Comprehensive Medical Assisting, Administrative and Clinical Competencies *(p. 824), by W. Lindh, M. S. Pooler, D. C. Tamparo, and J. U. Cerrato, 1998, Albany, NY: Delmar Publishers. Copyright 1998 by Delmar Publishers. Reprinted with permission.*

The lymphatic system is the last system in the body we discuss. Interstitial fluid is the fluid of this system. The lymphatic system drains the interstitial fluid from tissue spaces and returns it to the blood. The system also transports nutrients and oxygen and defends the body against infection by the interstitial fluid flowing around the body tissues. Lymph vessels run the course of the body similar to the blood vessels and transport the interstitial fluid.

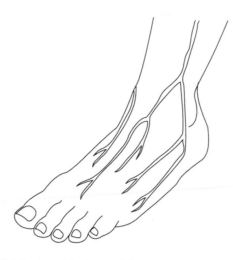

Figure 1.21 *Superficial veins of the legs and feet.*

REVIEW QUESTIONS

Multiple Choice

Choose the one best answer.

1. The formed elements make up about _____ percent of the whole blood volume.
   a. 30
   b. 60
   c. 55
   d. 45

2. The two components of blood found in a tube of blood drawn *without* anticoagulant are
   a. plasma and clot
   b. buffy coat and erythrocytes
   c. serum and buffy coat
   d. serum and clot

3. The buffy coat consists of
   a. leukocytes and thrombocytes
   b. leukocytes only
   c. erythrocytes and leukocytes
   d. leukocytes and plasma

4. The difference between plasma and serum is
   a. serum comes from anticoagulated blood; plasma does not
   b. plasma contains fibrinogen; serum does not
   c. serum contains fibrinogen; plasma does not
   d. plasma is only found inside the body

5. The fluid portion of the whole blood that contains fibrinogen is called
   a. buffy coat
   b. erythrocytes
   c. plasma
   d. serum

6. The fluid portion of blood after clotting has taken place is called
   a. buffy coat
   b. erythrocytes
   c. plasma
   d. serum

7. The main function of the circulatory system is to provide
   a. absorption
   b. elimination
   c. protection
   d. transportation

8. Blood returns to the heart from the lungs into the
   a. aorta
   b. left atrium
   c. pulmonary artery
   d. right atrium

9. The ventricles of the heart are principally responsible for
   a. lubrication
   b. portal circulation
   c. pumping blood
   d. receiving blood

10. Which of the following does *not* carry oxygenated blood?
    a. aorta
    b. pulmonary artery
    c. pulmonary vein
    d. all of the above

11. Which of the following is referred to as the "pacemaker" of the heart?
    a. AV node
    b. sinoatrial node
    c. bundle of His
    d. Purkinje's Fibers

12. What is the function of the coronary arteries?
    a. carry oxygenated blood back to the heart
    b. cause the blood to become oxygenated at the lungs
    c. supply oxygenated blood to the heart muscle
    d. none of the above

Critical Thinking

1. Explain the difference between serum and plasma samples.

2. What would you do if a patient wanted you to show him his test results?

3. How would you handle this situation? A terminal patient you are ready to collect blood from says, "I don't want my blood drawn. I'm just going to die anyway."

4. One of the coronary arteries becomes occluded. What could possibly happen to that patient?

BIBLIOGRAPHY

American Hospital Association. (1973, February). Procedures for examination and certification. Patient's Bill of Rights. *Hospitals, 47,* 41.

American Society of Clinical Pathologists. (1995). *Board of registry.* Chicago, Illinois.

Bissell, M., & Cosman, T. (1991, July). How ethical dilemmas induce stress. *Medical Laboratory Observer,* pp. 28–33.

Gylys, B. A., & Wedding, M. E. (1988). *Medical terminology: A systems approach.* Philadelphia: F. A. Davis.

Hoeltke, L. B. (1991, May). How internships eased our phlebotomist shortage. *Medical Laboratory Observer,* pp. 65–72.

Hoeltke, L. B. (1995). *Phlebotomy: The clinical laboratory manual series.* Albany, NY: Delmar.

Lindh, W., Pooler, M. S., Tamparo, C. D., & Cerrato, J. U. (1998). *Comprehensive medical assisting, administrative and clinical competencies.* Albany, NY: Delmar.

McCall, R. E., & Tankersley, C. M. (1993). *Phlebotomy essentials.* Philadelphia, J. B. Lippincott.

Mobley, R. C., & Simon, V. (1989). Coping with CLIA. *Diagnostics, 27*(9), 18–20.

Madison, S. K.: Patient self-determination act: Implications for long term care. *J Gerontol Nurs* 19:15–18, 1993.

National Committee for Clinical Laboratory Standards. (1998). *Procedures for the collection of diagnostic blood specimens by venipuncture,* (4th ed.). Approved Standard. NCCLS Document H3-A4. Villanova, PA: Author.

Sisk, F. A. (1991, July). Trends in regulation and reimbursement. *Medical Laboratory Observer,* pp. 49–55.

Snyder, J. R., & Senhauser, D. A. (1989). *Administration and supervision in laboratory medicine.* Philadelphia: J. B. Lippincott.

Steiner, J. W., Root, J. M., & Michel, R. L. (1995). The transformation of hospital laboratories: Why regionalization, consolidation, reengineering will lead laboratories into the 21st century. *AHA Hospital Technology Series.*

Tamparo, C. D., & Lindh, W. Q. (1992). *Therapeutic communications for allied health professions.* Albany, NY: Delmar.

Tilton, R. C., Balows, A., Hohnadel, D. C., & Reiss, R. F. (1992). *Clinical laboratory medicine.* St. Louis: Mosby-Year Book.

Trotto, N. E. (1991, October). Certification of laboratorians: An update. *Medical Laboratory Observer,* pp. 26–36.

Wedding, M. E., & Toenjes, S. A. (1992). *Medical laboratory procedures.* Philadelphia: F. A. Davis.

Chapter 2

SAFETY IN PHLEBOTOMY

O B J E C T I V E S

After studying this chapter, you should be able to:

1. Identify rules of safety that promote safety of the individual and patient.
2. Explain the principle and procedures for infection control.
3. Describe the proper handwashing technique and when to use it.
4. Explain the infection concept.
5. Explain the differences between disease-specific and category-specific isolation.
6. List the seven types of category-specific isolation.
7. Explain the purpose and scope of universal precautions.
8. State the five major tactics to reduce the risk of exposure to blood-borne pathogens.
9. Explain the concerns regarding latex gloves.
10. Describe precautionary measures and actions to be taken with accidental needle punctures.
11. Explain the purpose of Material Safety Data Sheets (MSDS).

KEY TERMS

Autoclave	Instrument for sterilizing that uses steam under pressure.
Autogenous Infection	Infection from one's own flora.
Biohazard	Anything that is potentially hazardous to humans, living organisms, or the environment.
Blood-Borne Pathogen	A pathogen that is spread by blood and body fluids containing blood. Typically, the pathogens are hepatitis and human immuno-deficiency virus (HIV).
Category-Specific Isolation	Isolation based on the category (strict, respiratory, etc.) of isolation.
Chemical Hazard	Any element, chemical compound, or mixture of elements and/or compounds that causes physical or health hazards.
Communicable Disease	Disease that is spread from person to person.
Disease-Specific Isolation	Isolation based on the type of disease infecting the patient.
Latex Allergy	An allergy to natural rubber latex. It is an allergy to the latex proteins that are released in the use of latex-containing products.
Local Infection	An infection affecting only one area of the body.
Nosocomial Infection	Infection as a result of a hospital or health facility stay.
Personal Protective Equipment (PPE)	Equipment that is used to protect the health care associate from exposure to blood and body fluids.
Sharps Container	Specially labeled puncture-resistant containers for the disposal of sharp items such as needles, scalpels, and syringes.
Systemic Infection	An infection affecting the entire body.

INFECTION CONTROL AND ISOLATION TECHNIQUES

Maintaining a safe working environment is of primary concern for all who work in or have exposure in the health care industry. Standards and procedures need to be formalized to protect the health care associate and the patient. These procedures are often established to protect the health care associate from being infected by the patient. The procedures also protect the patient from being infected by the health care associate or other patients. A patient who comes into a hospital and develops an infection as a result of the stay in the hospital is said to have obtained a **nosocomial infection.** A patient's infection can be a **local infection,** which is an infection restricted to one area of the body, or a **systemic infection,** which affects the entire body. If the organism that causes this infection and disease spreads from person to person, it is classified as a **communicable disease.** To understand the practices and standards used in a health care setting and how they work, you must understand the infection concept.

The spread of infection requires a source of infecting organisms, a susceptible host, and a means of transmission of the organism. Connecting these three factors are two different portals: a portal of exit from the source and a portal of entry into the susceptible host. What is created is a chain (Figure 2.1).

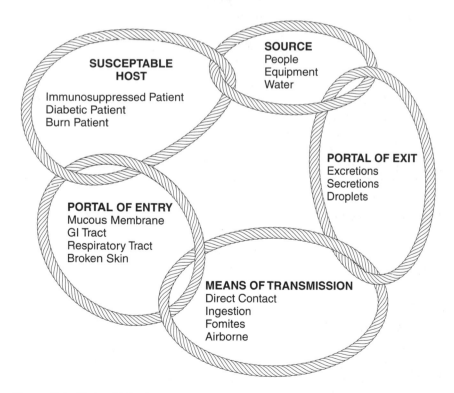

Figure 2.1 *Chain of infection.*

The source of an infection can be health care associates, other patients, or visitors. The source can be a person who has an active acute infection or who is carrying the infection and does not realize he or she has it. With the number of people contacting each other in a health care setting, the potential is great that the chain of infection can be started. The source and the host can be one and the same. The infection can come from the source's own flora (**autogenous infection**).

The susceptibility of the susceptible host to an infection varies greatly with the individual. A person who has never had chicken pox usually becomes infected when placed in contact with a source of chicken pox. A person who had chicken pox in childhood will not become infected. The key to the infection concept is that the host must be susceptible to the infecting organism. Age, disease, medication, and immunosuppressive agents often change a host's susceptibility. When a host's body defense mechanisms are weakened by chronic illness, AIDS (acquired immune deficiency syndrome), or by immunosuppressive agents, the host will contact many organisms that normally would not be infectious. Those organisms that we maintain as normal flora in the body, such as yeast or mycoplasma, are opportunistic and can cause infection when the conditions are right. Patients with HIV do not die of this disease but of opportunistic infections.

The means of transmission often follow one of four routes: contact, vehicle, airborne, or vectorborne. The contact transmission can either be direct, indirect, or droplet. Direct contact consists of a direct physical transfer of infective material from the source to the susceptible host—for example, a health care associate cleaning up after a patient and then, without handwashing between patients, transferring a contaminant to the next patient.

Indirect contact involves personal contact of the susceptible host to some type of object that has been contaminated such as instruments, bed linens, furniture, or shared bathrooms. Drainage from a source patient can be deposited on furniture. The susceptible host could touch the drainage, transferring it to an open wound or ingesting it, thus infecting the susceptible host.

Droplet contact is the transfer of the organism causing the infection to the nose, mouth, or eye by contact with the mucous membrane of a susceptible host. This is caused by the spread of the infectious droplets through the air by the source person coughing, sneezing, or talking. Because the droplets travel only a short distance, no more than 1 meter, this is still considered contact infection.

The vehicle route is the transfer of the disease-causing organism through contaminated items. Vehicles of disease can be as simple as contaminated food that results in food poisoning. Contaminated water is often the vehicle causing parasitic or cholera infections. Blood and body fluids are the vehicle transferring HIV or hepatitis to the host. The accidental needlestick and the blood of the patient (source) as the vehicle for infection of the phlebotomist (susceptible host) are of concern to each phlebotomist. The treatments for accidental needlesticks are covered later in the chapter (Procedure 2.4).

Airborne transmission is our concern in patients disseminating airborne droplets of infection as a result of coughing, sneezing, or talking and these droplets being inhaled or deposited on a susceptible host. The most commonly known disease transmitted by this means is tuberculosis.

Vector transmission is the transmission of a disease by insects. The most widely known vector-transmitted disease is mosquito-transmitted malaria. This is of little concern to hospitals in the United States but can be a major problem in developing tropical countries. Hospitals need to be concerned with flies, cockroaches, and other insects carrying microorganisms on their feet or other body parts. The insects can potentially be a problem to hospitals if they come in contact with infectious materials such as soiled dressings, bed pans, and so on.

Universal Precautions, or Standard Precautions

Universal precautions, also known as standard precautions, are blood and body fluid precautions that apply to all patients. Any patient has the potential to be infected with **blood-borne pathogens** such as hepatitis B virus (HBV) or HIV. Universal precautions assume that all blood and all body fluids of all patients are potentially infectious. Since it is impossible to know if a patient is infectious, the health care worker must treat all patients with the universal precautions for infection. Precaution guidelines have been established by the Centers for Disease Control (CDC) and the Occupational Safety and Health Administration (OSHA). These guidelines state that all patients are considered potentially infectious for hepatitis or HIV. All body substances must be treated as infectious. Universal precautions include a variety of body substances. The body substances linked to the transmission of hepatitis and HIV are blood, semen, vaginal secretions, cerebrospinal fluid, synovial fluid, pleural fluid, peritoneal fluid, pericardial fluid, amniotic fluid, human breast milk, and wound drainage. Universal precautions also apply to all tissue specimens before they are chemically fixed. Other fluids such as stool, urine, vomitus, and oral secretions are not included in universal precautions unless they contain visible blood. It is recommended that universal precautions be used when working with any body fluid. There is always the possibility that blood-borne pathogens are present in all body fluids even when blood is not visible. Following proper precautions with blood and body fluid can nearly eliminate the threat of a health care associate being infected with hepatitis or HIV by a patient.

Standard precautions combine many of the basic principles of universal precautions with techniques known as body substance isolation (BSI). This is a system that maintains that personal protective equipment must be worn for contact with all body fluids whether or not blood is visible. Standard precautions are to reduce the risk of transmission of microorganisms from both recognized and unrecognized sources of infection. Five main points must be followed in standard precautions:

- Wash hands when changing gloves and between patients.
- Wear gloves when likely to touch body substances, mucous membranes, or nonintact skin and during all blood drawing.
- Wear protective cover when clothing is likely to be soiled.
- Wear mask and eye protection in addition to a protective body cover when likely to be splashed with body substances.
- Place intact needle/syringe and sharps in designated sharps containers. Do not bend, break, or cut needles.

Six major tactics reduce the risk of exposure to blood-borne pathogens:

1. Engineering controls
2. Work practices
3. Personal protective equipment
4. Housekeeping
5. HBV vaccination
6. Isolation techniques

Engineering Controls

Engineering controls are physical and mechanical devices that are available to the health care associate to reduce or eliminate the potential to transfer infectious diseases. Examples of these are self-

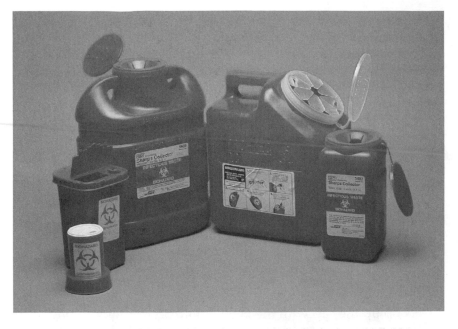

Figure 2.2 *Place used needles, point down, in puncture-proof sharps containers. Note. From* Comprehensive Medical Assisting, Administrative and Clinical Competencies *(p. 645), by W. Lindh, M. S. Pooler, D. C. Tamparo, and J. U. Cerrato, 1998, Albany, NY: Delmar Publishers. Copyright 1998 by Delmar Publishers. Reprinted with permission.*

sheathing needles; autoclaves, which steam sterilize contaminated materials; and puncture-proof **sharps containers** (Figure 2.2), which can be used for contaminated sharp objects such as needles and breakable contaminated objects such as glass blood collection tubes. These sharps containers are designed to be filled only to 80 percent of capacity to prevent accidental needle puncture by a health care associate overpacking the container. Blood collection tubes that are transported to the laboratory for testing must be placed in a self-sealing plastic bag. All specimens and containers should have a biohazard warning (Figure 2.8, later in this chapter), indicating the potential infectiousness of the contents.

Work Practice Controls

Work practice controls are practices that are incorporated into all health care associates' work habits to prevent the spread of infection. Handwashing is the single most important way to prevent the spread of infection. Hands must be washed after each patient contact or blood and body fluid exposure, even when gloves are used. Hands must be washed under running water with soap and vigorous rubbing. When rinsing the soap off, the water should flow from the wrists to the fingertips. Antiseptic nonwater hand cleaners or antiseptic towlettes are acceptable when running water is not available. These are temporary measures, and hands must be washed with soap and water as soon as possible.

Punctures with contaminated needles are a serious concern to all health care associates for transmission of infection and personal injury. The work practice of properly handling and disposing of contaminated sharps can eliminate a major source of occupationally acquired hepatitis or HIV. Contaminated needles and other contaminated sharps should not be recapped or removed unless no other feasible alternative exists. When no alternative exists, the recapping or removal must be accomplished with a mechanical device or a one-handed technique. The one-handed capping method is accomplished as follows:

1. Place the needle cap on a flat surface.
2. Scoop up the cap with the needle unit. Scooping with one hand prevents accidental needle puncture of the opposite hand.
3. Press the cap firmly onto the needle unit by pressing the cap on the flat surface.
4. Dispose of the recapped needle in a sharps container.

Eating, drinking, smoking, applying cosmetics or lip balm, and handling contact lenses are prohibited in work areas. Food and drink must not be kept in the same room where potentially infectious materials are present. Food and drink must be stored in refrigerators, freezers, and cabinets separate from potentially infectious materials. Food and drink must be consumed in a room separate from the work area. Before entering this room, all protective garments must be removed.

Personal Protective Equipment

Personal protective equipment (PPE) used by the phlebotomist may include masks, goggles, face shields, gowns, or gloves (Figures 2.3A & B). This equipment is used to protect the phlebotomist from infectious material contacting street clothes, skin, or mucous membranes. Employers must provide this equipment free of charge and must maintain and clean the equipment at no charge to the phlebotomist.

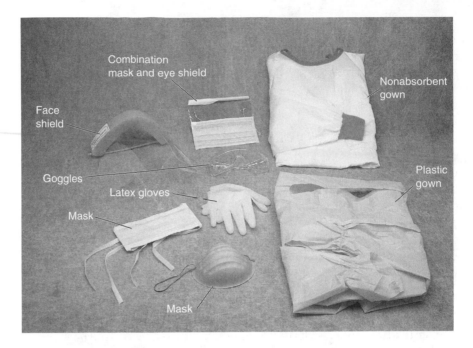

Figure 2.3A *Personal protective equipment (PPE). Note. From* Comprehensive Medical Assisting, Administrative and Clinical Competencies *(p. 66), by W. Lindh, M. S. Pooler, D. C. Tamparo, and J. U. Cerrato, 1998, Albany, NY: Delmar Publishers. Copyright 1998 by Delmar Publishers. Reprinted with permission.*

Housekeeping

Good housekeeping is the responsibility of all health care associates. Each facility has its own requirements for housekeeping. General rules for housekeeping involve cleaning up spills and decontaminating soiled areas immediately with a disinfectant such as 10 percent bleach that has been made up fresh daily. Broken glass should not be picked up with the hands. A brush and dustpan should be used.

Hepatitis B Vaccination

HBV vaccine must be available at no charge to the phlebotomist. The vaccine is administered in three injections over a period of six months. The complete series is effective for nine or more years in protecting the phlebotomist from contracting the disease or becoming a carrier.

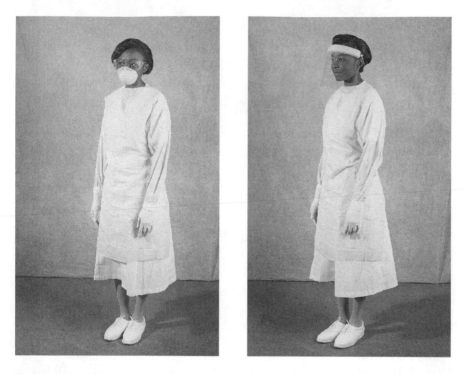

Figure 2.3B *Phlebotomist wearing personal protective equipment (PPE). Note. From* Comprehensive Medical Assisting, Administrative and Clinical Competencies *(p. 46), by W. Lindh, M. S. Pooler, D. C. Tamparo, and J. U. Cerrato, 1998, Albany, NY: Delmar Publishers. Copyright 1998 by Delmar Publishers. Reprinted with permission.*

Isolation Techniques

The means of transmission is the point where the health care team works to break the chain of infection. To do this, the patient is often placed in isolation. Isolation limits the amount of contact time a patient has to spread an infection. This isolation can be used to prevent the patient from spreading an infection to associates, other patients, or visitors. Isolation can also be used to prevent the spread of an infection to the patient. Handwashings between patients and using a new pair of gloves with each patient are the most critical behaviors used to prevent the spread of infection. Handwashing and gloves must be used with each patient contacted, even if the patient is not in isolation. Two basic types of isolation are recommended for patients: the category-specific system and the disease-specific system. To better understand how spread of infection can be prevented, let's look at the seven different types of category-specific isolation:

1. Strict isolation
2. Contact isolation
3. Respiratory isolation
4. Tuberculosis isolation
5. Drainage/secretion precautions
6. Enteric precautions
7. Protective or reverse isolation

Strict Isolation

A patient with a contagious disease such as chicken pox, diphtheria, or pneumonia is placed in strict isolation. The patient stays in a private room, and anyone entering that room is required to wear a mask, gown, and gloves. Only the phlebotomy equipment needed for that patient is to be taken into the room. The disposable equipment used to draw the patient, including the needle, gauze, needle holder, and tourniquet, must be left in the room. The only items to leave the room are the tubes that contain the blood sample.

Contact Isolation

A disease that is transmitted by direct contact with the patient requires the patient be placed in contact isolation. Scabies, caused by infestation with the mite *Sarcoptes scabei*, is an example of this type of disease. It is transmitted primarily through direct contact with the infested patient. Transmission occurs during sponge baths or when applying body lotion. Prevention of the spread of the infestation is best accomplished by avoiding direct contact until the patient has been treated. One treatment is usually curative to stop the spread, and then a second treatment at 7–10 days prevents a recurrence.

Respiratory Isolation

A patient with a disease transmitted through the air, such as mumps, pertussis, or rubella, may be placed in respiratory isolation. This isolation requires a private room with closed door. Anyone who is susceptible to the infection must wear a mask upon entering the room. Masks must not be worn around the neck to be slipped on whenever entering a respiratory isolation room. Discard the mask as you leave the room. A fresh mask must be used every twenty minutes. Once a mask has become moist from normal breathing, it is no longer effective.

Tuberculosis Isolation

Tuberculosis isolation, sometimes called AFB (acid-fast bacillus) isolation, is the isolation of the patient with tuberculosis. The isolation techniques are similar to respiratory isolation. Tuberculosis is an opportunistic type of disease. It infects the individual whose immune system has been weakened by some other disease process such as AIDS or simply old age. The tuberculosis then sets in because the body cannot fight the tuberculosis organism. With the increase in AIDS patients and more people living longer and in nursing homes, tuberculosis is on the rise.

Drainage/Secretion Precautions

Drainage/secretion precautions, sometimes called wound and skin precautions, are used for patients with open wounds. These are usually the result of abrasions, accidental skin cuts, surgery incisions, or bed sores that have become infected. The fluid that oozes from the wound contains the infection. The dressings that have absorbed the fluid and any fluid touched provide potential for transmission of that infection to the health care associate or to another patient. Gown, gloves, and mask are required for anyone who has direct contact with the wound, normally during dressing changes. The phlebotomist must always wear gloves, and only the equipment needed should be taken into the room. Upon leaving the room, take only the blood samples.

Enteric Precautions

Enteric precautions are for patients with severe diarrhea due to contagious bacteria such as *Salmonella, Shigella,* or *Vibrio cholerae.* These types of infections are transmitted by contact with the infected patient's feces. In the late nineteenth century, the outhouse toilet was the cause of much of the spread of the enteric infections. The outhouse was placed near the residence for convenience, and the water well was located only a few feet away. People did not realize they were continually reinfecting themselves until they moved the outhouse and the well went dry. Today's modern water purification and sewage treatment have nearly eliminated enteric infections. The last known cholera epidemic in the United States was in the late nineteenth century. Developing countries with inadequate or no sewage treatment are still experiencing enteric infections. Historically, cholera has been the cause of many epidemics and numerous deaths. Enteric infections today are caused primarily by *Salmonella* and *Shigella* species. These infections are caused primarily by eating improperly cooked meat, usually chicken. Infections of this type are less deadly but still require proper enteric precautions. Gown and gloves are required as in most other isolations, and only the equipment needed is to be taken into the room. When working with the patient, the phlebotomist should avoid contacting the feces of the patient.

Protective or Reverse Isolation

Many category-specific systems do not include protective or reverse isolation. This is because in most cases of category-specific isolation, the isolation is protecting the health care associate from the patient. With protective isolation, the isolation is protecting the patient from the health care associate. This type of isolation is no more or less important than any of the others and is specifically needed in many situations. Cancer patients who have reduced immunity and transplant patients are placed in protective or reverse isolation. These patients cannot fight off infection like normal individuals. The phlebotomist's slight runny nose may be an inconvenience to the phlebotomist but could be life threatening to a transplant patient. Instead of the phlebotomist trying to avoid being infected by the patient, the patient now needs to be protected from the phlebotomist. A mask, gown, and gloves are required. Your tray must stay outside the room so not to contaminate the patient. A clean evacuated tube holder and a new tourniquet must be used each time. Since the patient is not contagious, all equipment taken into the room can be removed.

Properly adhering to the universal precautions may be the biggest challenge facing health care workers today. AIDS, caused by HIV, has presented a great challenge because there is no known cure. HIV also challenges us because of the complex emotional, social, and moral issues it involves. Many health care workers have had to overcome a fear of HIV and explain to their families their decision to continue working where HIV is a threat.

These different types of isolation are the key to **category-specific isolation.** All isolation procedures fall into a category according to the type of isolations previously described: strict isolation, respiratory isolation, and so on. There is some compromise in this type of isolation. Certain precautions that are necessary for the majority of diseases in a certain category may not be necessary for others. The recommendations generally incorporate the more rigorous precautions. It is safer to "overisolate" than "underisolate." A specific color-coded card or sign is placed on the door to indicate the type of isolation precautions to be used (Figure 2.4).

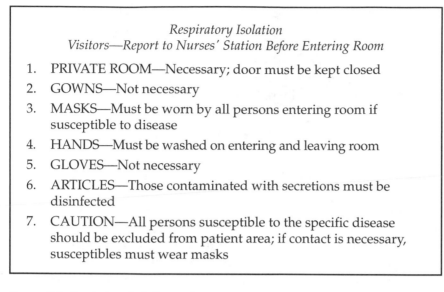

Respiratory Isolation
Visitors—Report to Nurses' Station Before Entering Room

1.   PRIVATE ROOM—Necessary; door must be kept closed
2.   GOWNS—Not necessary
3.   MASKS—Must be worn by all persons entering room if susceptible to disease
4.   HANDS—Must be washed on entering and leaving room
5.   GLOVES—Not necessary
6.   ARTICLES—Those contaminated with secretions must be disinfected
7.   CAUTION—All persons susceptible to the specific disease should be excluded from patient area; if contact is necessary, susceptibles must wear masks

Figure 2.4 *Respiratory isolation card.*

Disease-specific isolation precautions have been established to overcome the compromises in category-specific isolation. Disease-specific isolation uses a listing of different diseases and lists yes or no answers to questions whether a private room, masks, gowns or gloves are needed for each disease. The list is consulted for each patient. Then a card is attached to the patient's door listing the required isolation precautions (Figure 2.5). Patients infected with the same organism may share a room. For some diseases or conditions, a private room is necessary if the patient's hygiene is poor. Patients with poor hygiene (infants, children, or altered mental status) can contaminate their environment with infective material or share contaminated articles with other patients. For some diseases a mask is necessary only for those who get close.

Most health care organizations are using a blend of universal precautions and category-specific or disease-specific isolation. Patients who have a known infectious disease are placed in the proper isolation. All other patients are treated according to universal precautions.

The largest problem with isolation procedures is the health care associate not fully complying with the proper isolation procedures. If the health care associate takes shortcuts in the procedure, the potential is there for a transmission of infection. When entering a patient's room, the protective equipment must be used

Visitors—Report to Nurses' Station Before Entering Room

1. Private room indicated?   ___ No
                               ___ Yes

2. Masks indicated?   ___ No
                        ___ Yes for those close to patient
                        ___ Yes for all persons entering room

3. Gowns indicated?   ___ No
                        ___ Yes if soiling is likely
                        ___ Yes for all persons entering room

4. Gloves indicated?   ___ No
                         ___ Yes for touching infective material
                         ___ Yes for all persons entering room

5. Special precautions indicated   ___ No
    for handling blood?   ___ Yes

6. Hands must be washed after touching the patient or potentially contaminated articles and before taking care of another patient.

7. Articles contaminated with _____ should be red-bagged
                                  infective material(s)
    and discarded or red-bagged and labeled before being sent for decontamination and reprocessing.

INSTRUCTIONS

1. On the table Disease-Specific Isolation precautions, locate the disease for which isolation precautions are indicated.

2. Write disease in blank space here:

3. Determine if a private room is indicated. In general, patients infected with the same organism may share a room. For some diseases or conditions, a private room is indicated if patient hygiene is poor (infants, children, altered mental status, etc.). A patient with poor hygiene does not wash hands after touching infective material (feces, purulent drainage, or secretions), contaminates the environment with infective material, or shares contaminated articles with other patients.

4. Place a check mark beside the indicated precautions on front of card.

5. Cross through precautions that are not indicated.

6. Write infective material in blank space in item 7 on front of card.

Figure 2.5 *Disease-specific isolation.*

correctly and isolation methods performed according to the established standards, or the health care associate will be at risk. Universal precautions and isolation precautions have the following equipment and techniques in common.

Handwashing

Handwashing is the single most important way to prevent the spread of infection. Hands must be washed after each patient contact even when gloves are used. Disinfectant nonwater hand cleaners are only used when running water is not available. To further protect yourself, you should wash hands before and after eating and before and after using the restroom.

PROCEDURE 2.1

MEDICAL ASEPSIS HANDWASHING

Principle:

To clean the hands and reduce the number of organisms on the hands and wrists. The purpose is to decrease the transfer of organisms from a source to a susceptible host.

Materials:

Sink with running water, preferably foot-operated controls.
Soap from a foot-operated container or a pump container. Bar soap is discouraged.
Disposable paper towel.
Nail stick and/or brush.

Procedure:

1. Remove all rings, watches, and so on to prevent the jewelry from harboring microorganisms.
2. Have disposable towels ready so that you do not have to touch the towel dispenser.
3. Stand back from the sink so that you or your clothing do not touch the sink.
4. Turn on the water with the foot pedal or with a disposable towel if not foot controlled. Temperature should be lukewarm (Figure 2.6A).

continues

PROCEDURE 2.1   *continued*

5. Wet hands under the running water. Be careful to not touch the sides of the sink (Figure 2.6B).

6. Apply soap, and lather well. The lather and scrubbing action will remove dirt and dead skin. Scrub between fingers and around fingernails (Figure 2.6C). Use a nailstick and a brush during the first handwashing of each day or when your hands become excessively soiled (Figures 2.6D & E).

7. Rinse hands with the water flowing downward off the fingertips. This will rinse the contaminated water off the fingertips and not onto the forearms (Figure 2.6F).

8. Complete the washing process again if this is the first handwashing of the day. (Repeat steps 6 and 7.)

9. Dry hands and wrists with the disposable towels.

10. Turn off water with the disposable towels if the sink is not foot controlled.

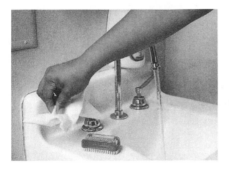

Figure 2.6A *Prepare towels for use; turn on water.*

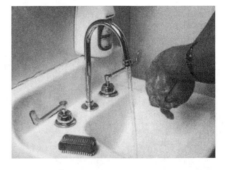

Figure 2.6B *Wet hands under the running water.*

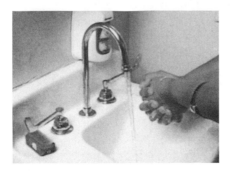

Figure 2.6C *Apply soap and lather well.*

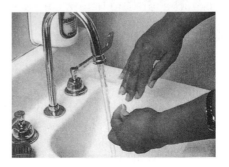

Figure 2.6D *Use a nailstick under the fingernails.*

continues

PROCEDURE 2.1 *continued*

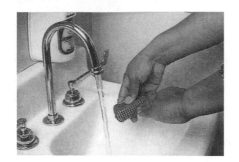

Figure 2.6E *Use a brush to clean around fingernails.*

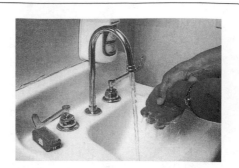

Figure 2.6F *Rinse hands with water flowing downward off hands and fingertips.*

Figure 2.6 *Medical asepsis handwashing. Note. From* Comprehensive Medical Assisting, Administrative and Clinical Competencies *(p. 376–377), by W. Lindh, M. S. Pooler, D. C. Tamparo, and J. U. Cerrato, 1998, Albany, NY: Delmar Publishers. Copyright 1998 by Delmar Publishers. Reprinted with permission.*

Private Room

A private room reduces the possibility of transmission of infection by separating the diseased patient from other patients and health care associates. The room should ideally have an anteroom where anyone entering or leaving the room can wash their hands and change protective garments.

Masks

Masks are used to prevent the transmission of infectious agents through the air. The health care associate should wear a mask when entering the room of a respiratory isolation patient. Paper masks are the most economical and efficient for the work of a phlebotomist. Fluid-proof masks are available for work conditions in which spattering of body fluids is likely. The mask should be worn once and then discarded in an appropriate container. The mask should never be worn around the neck and moved up to cover the nose and mouth as you enter another room. As noted, masks are no longer effective once they become moist from breathing, so they should never be used longer than 15–20 minutes. A patient in protective isolation needs to wear a mask during transport to another location. It is impossible to have everyone in the hospital hallways put on a mask, so the patient wears a mask to be protected from inhaling anything potentially infectious.

Goggles/Face Shields

Goggles or face shields are needed when there is the potential for splattering of blood or body fluids. A face shield should be constructed so that the eyes and mouth are protected. The shield should cover the face, preventing any splattering from getting into the mouth or eyes by entering through the sides or bottom of the shield. The shield can be a face shield the health care associate wears, or it can be a free-standing or movable shield that positions between the health care associate and the work.

Goggles can also be used for eye protection from splattering. Glasses can be used as long as side shields are attached to prevent blood or body fluids from entering from the side. Whenever a procedure warrants the use of goggles to protect the health care associate, a mask must also be used to prevent splattering from entering the mouth. Masks are available that have an eye shield attached to protect both the mouth and eyes.

Gowns

Gowns are necessary when soiling of your clothes is possible while taking care of patients. The gowns should be fluid resistant to prevent any blood or body fluids from soaking through the gown and getting on the health care associate. Gowns are also used in caring for patients who have infections that can be transmitted easily, such as varicella (chicken pox). Gowns should be used only once and then disposed of in the appropriate receptacle. Removal of the gown should be from the inside out. The gown is pulled down off the shoulders, slid down the arms, and folded with the inside out before final removal.

Gloves

There are three reasons gloves should be worn. First, sterile gloves prevent health care associates from transmitting their own microflora to the patient, such as during surgery or wound cleansing. Second, gloves prevent the transmission of microorganisms from one patient to another. Third, gloves prevent the associate from becoming infected with what is infecting the patient. Always remove gloves according to the following procedure:

PROCEDURE 2.2

REMOVING CONTAMINATED GLOVES

Principle:

To remove gloves after use to avoid contamination of the health care associate. The purpose is to decrease the transfer of organisms from a source to a susceptible host.

Materials:

Biohazard waste container.

Procedure:

1. Hold hands out in front away from the body.
2. Grasp the palm of one hand, and pull down on the glove to pull the glove inside out. A right-handed person would naturally pull the palm of the left hand (Figures 2.7A–D).
3. The hand still having the glove on should then hold the removed glove (Figure 2.7E).
4. Insert two fingers of the ungloved hand under the cuff of the glove of the other hand (Figure 2.7F).

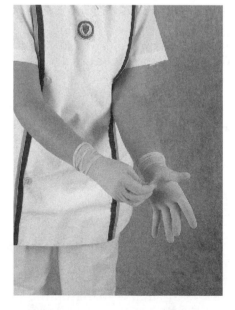

Figure 2.7A *Grasp the palm of the used glove.*

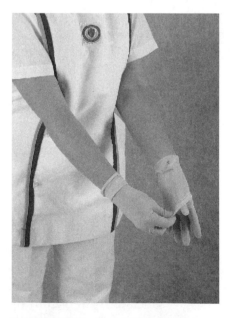

Figure 2.7B *Begin removing the first glove.*

continues

PROCEDURE 2.2 *continued*

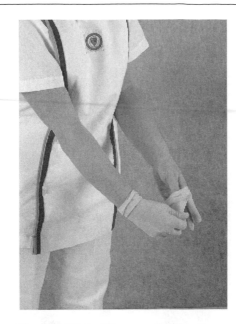

Figure 2.7C *Pull down on the glove to pull it inside out.*

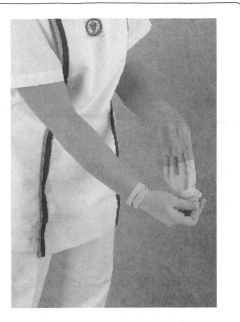

Figure 2.7D *Pull the left glove into the right glove.*

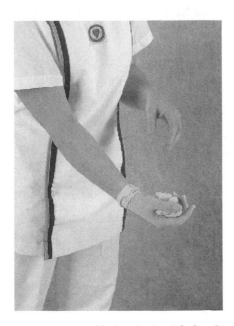

Figure 2.7E *Hold glove in the right hand.*

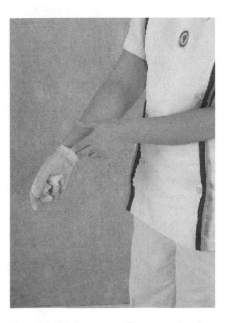

Figure 2.7F *Insert two fingers under the cuff of the other glove.*

continues

PROCEDURE 2.2 *continued*

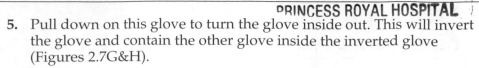

5. Pull down on this glove to turn the glove inside out. This will invert the glove and contain the other glove inside the inverted glove (Figures 2.7G&H).

6. Dispose of the gloves into a biohazard container (Figure 2.7I).

7. Wash hands with running water.

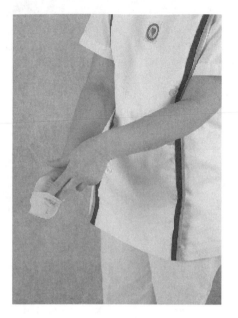

Figure 2.7G *Use the two ungloved fingers to pull the glove inside out.*

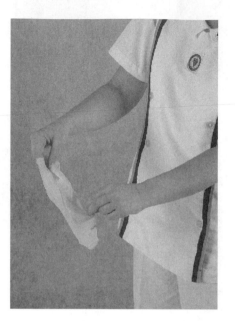

Figure 2.7H *One glove is now inside of the other.*

Figure 2.7 *Removing contaminated gloves. Note. From* Comprehensive Medical Assisting, Administrative and Clinical Competencies *(p. 380), by W. Lindh, M. S. Pooler, D. C. Tamparo, and J. U. Cerrato, 1998, Albany, NY: Delmar Publishers. Copyright 1998 by Delmar Publishers. Reprinted with permission.*

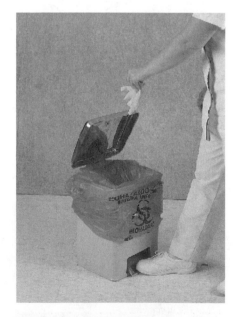

Figure 2.7I *Dispose of gloves in a biohazard container.*

Bagging of Articles

Used articles must be enclosed in an impervious bag before they are removed from the isolation room. This bagging prevents exposure of associates to the contaminated materials. A double-bagging method is used. The articles bagged in the isolation room are sealed, and the bag is dropped into a bag held by an individual outside the room. The double-bagged articles can then be transported without the possibility of contamination. In reality, two associates are usually not available, and a modification of the double-bagging technique is necessary. This is further explained in the following isolation procedure (Procedure 2.3).

The collection of blood from a patient in an isolation room follows a specific procedure. This procedure is the easiest when two people are available and one individual can receive the tubes of blood in a zip-lock transport bag at the door. The following procedure has been written with the reality that usually the phlebotomist is working alone.

PROCEDURE 2.3

BLOOD COLLECTION IN AN ISOLATION ROOM

Principle:

To protect the patient or health care associate from the transmission of disease-causing organisms.

Materials:

Blood collection equipment as required per collection technique.

Procedure:

1. Remove all rings, watches, and so on.
2. Prepare to take only essential items into the isolation room. Do not take your tray into the isolation room.
3. Check the isolation card on the door for isolation instructions. The card should have specific information regarding the isolation attire needed.
4. When entering the anteroom, remove three paper towels from the paper towel dispenser. Spread the paper towels open, and lay one on top of the other. Place the phlebotomy equipment in the center of the top towel.

continues

5. Wash your hands with soap and water after entering the anteroom. Rinse by letting the water run from the wrists to the fingertips.

6. Dress according to the isolation card instructions. First put on the gown, being careful it does not touch the floor. Put on the mask next, making certain it covers the nose and the mouth.

7. Check to see if a tourniquet and evacuated tube holder are already in the room. Carry the towels with the equipment you will need into the patient's room.

8. Check the patient's armband, and draw the specimens according the required procedure.

9. Discard needles, syringes, and all contaminated equipment in the sharps container. Leave the evacuated tube holder and tourniquet in the room.

10. Open a new alcohol wipe, and wipe off the outside of each tube and stopper. Before laying down the cleaned tubes, discard the top paper towel. Now place the tubes on the second towel. Pick up the second towel with the tubes wrapped inside and discard the third (bottom) towel.

11. Carry the tubes and towel into the anteroom.

12. Label tubes.

13. Place tubes, discarding the last towel, in a zip-lock specimen transport bag.

14. Remove isolation attire in the following order:
    First: Remove your face mask, touching only the strings.
    Second: Remove your gown by touching only the inside. Fold the gown so the inside of the gown now faces out and place the gown in the hamper.
    Third: Remove gloves according to Procedure 2.2.

15. Wash hands thoroughly.

OCCUPATIONAL SAFETY AND HEALTH ADMINISTRATION STANDARDS

The Occupational Safety and Health Administration (OSHA) is an agency of the federal government that investigates the possibility of unsafe practices in the work environment. OSHA was a result of the Occupational Safety and Health Act of 1970. The goal of OSHA is to promote safety for health care workers and their environment. This is done by the following OSHA functions:

- Develop and promote health and safety standards for all occupations.
- Develop and issue regulations.
- Determine the level of compliance of health and safety regulations.
- Level fines for noncompliance with health and safety regulations.

OSHA is notorious for leveling fines against hospitals for noncompliance with federal regulations. OSHA inspectors usually do not travel from hospital to hospital looking for noncompliance. They are usually invited by an associate who feels he or she is working under unsafe conditions. Once they are in the hospital, the inspectors investigate more than just the area of complaint. They usually investigate the safety status of the entire hospital. This process can sometimes take months to complete. The investigation includes inspection of records, watching work performance, and associate and management interviews. The interviews are the most difficult part because the inspectors are trying to prove that the associates at all levels know what management and the records have claimed to have told them.

The rules and regulations that health care institutions must comply with are published in a government publication called the *Federal Register.* In December 1991, a revision of the regulations created strict standards that must be maintained by all health care institutions. After a six-month introduction period, all rules and regulations had to be in compliance by July 6, 1992. These regulations override any other guidelines issued by any other agency, either government or private.

The entire regulations encompass hundreds of pages and include important points for anyone in contact with patients, blood, and body fluids. The OSHA regulations encompass three plans: an exposure control plan, engineering control plan, and work practice control plan. Every health care facility should have an exposure control plan. This plan will outline health and safety guidelines for that health care facility to protect the worker. The plan will incorporate the five tactics to reduce blood-borne pathogen exposure: engineering controls, work practices, personal protective equipment, housekeeping, and HBV vaccination availability.

Exposure Control Plan

Employers having employee(s) with occupational exposure to potentially infectious materials must establish a written exposure control plan designed to eliminate or minimize employee exposure. This plan should be accessible to OSHA inspectors and employees and must be reviewed and updated annually. Each job is classified according to what type of occupational exposure could occur. A method of implementation of the program and a method of communication of the potential hazards to all employees must be in place.

Needles and Sharps

Contaminated needles and other contaminated sharps should not be recapped, bent, cut, or broken. Contaminated needles and other contaminated sharps should not be recapped or removed unless no other feasible alternative exists. When no other alternative exists, the recapping or removal must be accomplished with a mechanical device or a one-handed technique. The one-handed capping method is accomplished as follows:

1. Place the needle cap on a flat surface.
2. Scoop up the cap with the needle unit. Scooping with one hand prevents accidental needle puncture of the opposite hand.
3. Press the cap firmly onto the needle unit by pressing the cap on the flat surface.
4. Dispose of the recapped needle in a sharps container.

All needles and sharps must be placed in containers that are puncture resistant, leakproof, and labeled or color coded as **biohazard.**

The biohazard labels must be fluorescent orange or orange-red with lettering or symbols in a contrasting color (Figure 2.8). The warning labels must also be affixed to containers of regulated waste and refrigerators or freezers containing blood or other potentially infectious material. Any containers used for transport or storage must also be labeled, and such containers must be of a sealed and leakproof construction. Blood is transported in a leakproof container. This includes the phlebotomist transporting blood from the patient to the laboratory. The required mode of transport is in a container, so if the tube containing the blood should break, the blood would be contained in the transport container. A number of containers can fill this requirement for transport of specimens within the health care setting. Zip-lock bags are the most convenient, but Tupperware-type containers, paint buckets, or plastic buckets with a sealable lid can also be used. For transport of potentially infectious materials through the mail, a separate set of standards is used by the postal service.

Figure 2.8 *Universal biohazard symbol.*

Laboratory Techniques

All procedures involving blood or potentially infectious materials are to be performed to minimize splashing, splattering, or generation of droplets. The Hemogard-type blood tube as described in Chapter 3 was created to meet this requirement.

Mouth pipetting or mouth suctioning of any potentially infectious material is prohibited. Pens, pencils, and fingers should not be placed in the mouth.

While working with any potentially infectious material, the health care associate must wear gloves and protective clothing. This standard must also be followed by all phlebotomists. The protective equipment is to be supplied at no cost to the associate. Any laundering or disposal of the protective equipment is to be done by the health care institution.

The OSHA regulations are for the protection of the associate in the health care setting. Often they seem to be written in ways to make the job slower and more tedious. They are simply common-sense items that prevent the health care associate from acquiring a job-related injury or infection.

Material Safety Data Sheets

The clinical laboratory contains a large array of hazards ranging from the previously mentioned biological hazards to chemical and electrical hazards. The awareness of **chemical hazards** has been the focus of OSHA since 1987, when Material Safety Data Sheets (MSDS) were first introduced. The MSDS are information sheets that must be kept on file and that indicate the hazards of the chemicals used in each section of the laboratory. Chemicals used in the laboratory must also contain labels with the identity of the chemical and show warnings appropriate for employee protection. This Hazard Communication Act is better known as the "right to know" law.

This act requires that the MSDS be readily accessible to all associates. New associates must receive training in the chemical hazards before starting work and have this training documented. A documented annual retraining of each associate must also occur.

Hazard Identification

Hazards can be identified on the container by a hazard emblem designed by the National Fire Protection Association (Figure 2.9). The system consists of a diamond-shaped diagram further subdivided into smaller diamonds. Health hazards are identified at the left, flammability at the top, and reactivity at the right. The bottom space is used to identify other hazards or to alert fire-fighting personnel to the possible hazard of using water. The hazards are identified by color: blue for health hazards, red for flammability, and yellow for reactivity. The diamonds are identified by number on a scale of 0–4 to indicate the severity of the hazard. Containers labeled "0" show no unusual hazard and those labeled "4" are extremely dangerous.

Fire Safety

Fire safety is taught periodically by each institution. Fire escape routes and your responsibility in a fire are specific for the institution. Fire extinguishers used in a fire are classified according to the type of fire they are to be used on.

Class A fire extinguishers are used on Class A fires, which include foam, loaded-stream, and multipurpose dry chemical extinguishers. Class A includes fires of ordinary combustible materials in the laboratory such as wood, plastics, and paper; that is, elements that require the cooling action of water to extinguish the fire.

Class B includes fires of flammable liquids and gases; that is, elements that require the blockage of oxygen from the fire to extinguish it. Class B fire extinguishers include carbon dioxide, dry chemical, foam, and loaded-stream extinguishers.

Fires in energized electrical equipment are classified as Class C fires. The use of nonconductive media is needed to prevent electrical shock when putting out the fire. Class C fire extinguishers

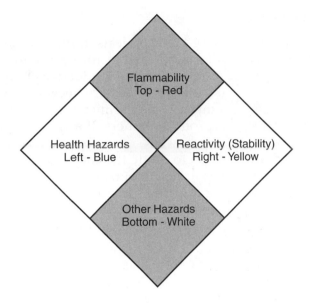

Figure 2.9 *Hazard identification system.*

include carbon dioxide, and dry chemical extinguishers. The carbon dioxide extinguisher seems to be the best universal fire extinguisher for the laboratory around computer equipment. It puts out the fire without damaging the computer circuits.

Class D includes fires of combustible and reactive metals such as sodium, potassium, magnesium, and lithium. These fires pose special problems, since explosion and spreading can easily occur. Class D fire extinguishers used on these types of fires contain a dry powder medium that does not react or combine with the burning materials.

Most fire extinguishers found in the laboratory are of a universal ABC-type fire extinguisher. The laboratory generally does not have metals that would require the use of a Class D fire extinguisher.

If there is a fire, the National Fire Protection Association's key word for action is **"RACE."**

R = **Rescue** anyone in danger.

A = Sound the **Alarm.**

C = **Contain** the fire by closing doors or windows.

E = **Extinguish/Evacuate.** Extinguish the fire if possible; if the fire is too large to extinguish, start to evacuate anyone in the fire's path.

Chemical Exposure

The phlebotomist is exposed to chemicals in the laboratory. These can be acids or alkalis that are harmful when in contact with the skin, eyes, or mouth. Goggles, protective clothing, and working behind special chemical hoods are necessary when using or dispensing chemicals. The chemicals should be transported in special shatterproof containers. If a spill or splatter does occur, eye wash and showers should be near. The shower dumps water on the person to dilute the chemical. The eye wash flows water onto the eye surface. A person using the eye wash will need help in holding the eye open and removing any contact lens that might be in the eye. The eye should be washed continuously for fifteen minutes and then the person taken for treatment.

Radiation Exposure

Phlebotomists are exposed to radiation. Radiation is present in nuclear medicine, radiology, the radioimmunoassay section of the chemistry laboratory, and patients with radioactive implants. Whenever phlebotomists encounter the radiation hazard symbol (Figure 2.10), they must be aware of the institution's radiation safety procedures. Most procedures limit the exposure by limiting the time the phlebotomist is exposed. The phlebotomist may need to be shielded with a special apron or cover gown. The only other method of protection is staying away from the radiation hazard.

Latex Allergy

Latex, which is made from the natural rubber of trees, can be found in many household and health care products. Balloons, toys, garden hoses, rubber gloves, tourniquets, intravenous tubing, blood pressure cuffs, and bandages are a few of the products that can contain latex. **Latex allergy** has been on the increase, as there is more exposure to latex products. Phlebotomists are at high risk due to their constant exposure to latex tourniquets and latex gloves.

Reactions to latex can vary with the individual. The reaction to the skin can be itchy irritation to redness and swelling that progresses to thickened skin, pimples, or skin blisters that ooze. This is the typical less serious type IV allergy to latex due to contact dermatitis. The symptoms begin 24–72 hours after

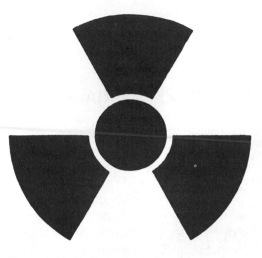

Figure 2.10 *Radiation hazard symbol.*

exposure and can continue for several days. With each additional exposure, the symptoms become more advanced.

Type I latex allergy is the more serious form of the allergy. This is an immunological reaction that is caused by the penetration of the natural latex proteins into the skin. These proteins cause a production of antibodies to latex, which increases with each subsequent exposure. As the allergy becomes more severe, the symptoms may include nausea, low blood pressure, and respiratory distress. If the latex allergen is introduced directly into the blood, then anaphylactic shock is possible. This can be life threatening.

To prevent allergic reactions from occurring, exposure to latex must be eliminated. There is no cure for latex allergy, only prevention of exposure. This prevention of exposure is not only for the phlebotomist but also for the patient. If the phlebotomist has a latex allergy, the phlebotomist must not work with latex gloves or tourniquets. If the patient has a latex allergy, the phlebotomist must avoid any type of latex contact to the patient. This includes the tourniquet, latex gloves, blood pressure cuffs, or bandage.

Latex allergies do not always come in the form of direct contact to the skin. The powder in the gloves disperses the latex into the air, and then the phlebotomist or the patient inhales the powder, causing a respiratory reaction. A less serious form of powder allergy is to get the powder in the eyes, and the eyes become irritated and swollen. Most health care providers are switching to powder-free gloves to avoid problems.

DISPOSAL OF USED MATERIALS

The disposal of potentially infectious materials is controlled by state laws more than by federal regulations. General requirements are standard in most states. A health care institution cannot just set the trash out on the curb and wait for the garbage truck to pick it up.

There are two requirements of disposal of medical waste. The first is to alter the product so no one can remove used needles or syringes or other devices for their own personal use or be injured by an exposed sharp. Second, the waste must be rendered noninfectious so that people handling the waste will not become infected and the environment will not be contaminated. There are three methods of disposal that meet these requirements: (1) incineration, (2) chemical treatment, and (3) autoclave.

The most common method of disposal of infectious waste is to incinerate it. The waste is burned to an ash and then the ash is taken to the municipal disposal area. This method kills any potentially infectious organisms and makes the items within the waste nonusable. Most large hospitals have incinerators to destroy waste and generate steam as a by-product.

If a health care institution does not have its own incinerator, it must rely on a commercial medical waste handler to dispose of the waste. The commercial medical waste handler will charge the health care institution by the weight of the waste. It is critical that only hazardous waste is placed in the biohazard waste receptacle. Items such as the paper towels you dry your hands with after washing should be not placed in the biohazard waste. Any increase in weight also increases the cost of disposal.

The commercial waste handler often uses the chemical treatment method of waste destruction. This method consists of grinding or chopping the waste into small pellets and then treating the pellets with a disinfectant chemical to kill any infectious organisms. The grinding process renders the waste unusable, while the disinfectant permits the waste to be sent to the municipal disposal site.

The autoclave method can be used in small operations where only a small amount of waste is generated. The **autoclave** is similar to a pressure cooker. The waste material is placed in the autoclave, and then the door is sealed shut. The door looks similar to a miniature submarine door with a wheel in the center. Once sealed, the autoclave is injected with steam to "cook" the waste under pressure. The plastics in the waste melt together to make the waste useless, and the infectious organisms are killed. Like the other methods, the waste can now be disposed of as normal trash.

Disposal of contaminated waste can be expensive. If you are working for a small office, the contaminated waste must be separated from general household-type trash. Too often, noninfectious materials are thrown into the infectious waste and then must go through special processing. Special containers should be established for infectious waste, just as there are special disposal containers for sharps.

IMPORTANCE OF FOLLOWING SAFETY GUIDELINES

The importance of following safety guidelines are twofold: the patient's safety and the phlebotomist's safety. The patient does not want to come into the health care setting and acquire a nosocomial infection. The phlebotomist does not want to come to work and acquire an infection from patient contact. That is the basic reason safety guidelines have been established.

OSHA has helped health care institutions to realize the importance of following their safety rules and regulations. If infractions are found during an OSHA inspection, the OSHA inspector can charge the health care setting up to $7,000 per infraction. For example, if the OSHA inspector watched the phlebotomists drawing blood and on seven occasions the phlebotomists did not wear gloves, the health care setting could be fined $49,000. Taking shortcuts in safety not only puts the phlebotomist at risk for infection, it can also cost the employer a considerable amount of money. By being notorious for large fines, OSHA has been able to enforce strong compliance to their rules and regulations.

Patients are also aware of specific safety rules and regulations. Patients often ask if that is a new needle, or if those are clean gloves. Patients who develop an infection due to negligence on the part of the health care associate's not following safety rules can sue. These lawsuits can take years to settle and often cost phenomenal amounts.

More important than money is the health care associate's own health. The special procedure detailed in Procedure 2.4 must be followed after any exposure from needlestick or splash:

RESPONSE TO ACCIDENTAL BIOHAZARD EXPOSURE

Principle:

An accidental biohazard exposure is defined as any exposure of the health care associate to blood, body fluids, or tissues. The exposure can be to the nonintact skin, mucous surface, or conjunctiva. This exposure may be via splash, splatter, needlestick, abrasion, or laceration. If an incident occurs, the associate must follow this procedure.

Materials:

Equipment to collect blood samples for testing.

Proper documents for documentation of circumstances about incident.

Procedure:

1. Immediately wash the exposed area with soap and water. If the mouth area is exposed, rinse with water or mouthwash. If eyes are exposed, flush with large amounts of warm water.
2. Report the incident to your supervisor immediately. Be prepared with information about the circumstances of the exposure. The supervisor will be required to document all information about the incident.
   a. What patient did the body fluid come from during the exposure? What is the source of the body fluid if known?
   b. What area of your body was exposed? For example, eyes? Right index finger punctured with a needle?
   c. Severity of the exposure.
   d. Exact time and date of the exposure.
3. The exposed associate must be tested for HIV and HBV only if the associate gives consent. An associate may refuse to have blood drawn or have blood drawn and stored for ninety days while the associate decides if the blood should be tested.
4. The source individual's blood is tested for HIV and HBV if the source individual gives consent.
5. The associate may be given the results of the testing if not prohibited by law.
6. If the source patient refuses testing, is HIV or HBV positive, or is in a high-risk category, the associate may elect to receive prophylaxis treatment as outlined in step 8. The associate is counseled and given follow-up testing at periodic intervals.

continues

7. All exposed associates are counseled to be alert for viral symptoms for twelve weeks after exposure.

8. ZDV (zidovudine) is offered as a prophylaxis to associates after an exposure such as a contaminated needle or deep-injury laceration. ZDV is sometimes used in combination with a protease inhibitor such as indinavir (IDV) to create a "cocktail" for high-risk exposures. Prophylactic treatment should be considered if (a) there has been an exposure to an HIV-positive patient; (b) the patient has a high-risk history (drug abuse); or (c) the source is unknown (needle in trash, etc.).

REVIEW QUESTIONS

Multiple Choice

Choose the one best answer.

1. The single most important way to prevent the spread of infection in a hospital or other facility is
   a. gowning and gloving
   b. handwashing
   c. always wearing masks
   d. avoiding breathing on patients

2. All of the following are components in the chain of infection *except*
   a. source
   b. mode of transportation
   c. poor isolation technique
   d. susceptible host

3. When a patient develops an infection during hospitalization that was not present upon admission, the infection is classified as
   a. nosocomial
   b. communicable
   c. infectious
   d. unavoidable

4. The primary purpose of infection control is to
   a. determine the source of communicable disease
   b. isolate patients from other patients and visitors
   c. protect the patient from outside contamination
   d. prevent the spread of infection within hospitals and other health care facilities

5. A potential source of infectious material from a patient in protective isolation includes
   a. feces
   b. none (the phlebotomist is considered a potential source of infection to the patient)
   c. urine
   d. blood

6. Aerosols can be produced by
   a. centrifuging open serum tubes
   b. popping open blood containers
   c. pouring off a serum sample
   d. all of the above

7. When coming into contact with patients under protective isolation, it is necessary to wear
   a. mask
   b. gloves
   c. gown
   d. all of the above

8. Universal precautions policy states that if there is a possibility of coming into contact with a patient's blood or any other body fluid you must wear
   a. a gown
   b. goggles
   c. gloves
   d. nothing, but wash hands immediately

9. According to universal precautions, blood and body fluids from which group are considered biohazardous?

   a. IV drug users
   b. homosexuals
   c. HIV-positive patients
   d. all blood and body fluids

10. Under universal precautions, all used needles are to be disposed of in the following manner
    a. recapped
    b. discarded intact
    c. bent
    d. broken or cut off

Critical Thinking

1. You walk into a patient's room to draw blood and notice a fire in the patient's wastebasket. What would you do?

2. After drawing blood from a patient, you puncture yourself in the left thumb. What actions should you immediately take?

3. Observe someone performing a venipuncture. What personal protective equipment did they use in the procedure? Was there any equipment that they should have used and did not use?

4. You are ready to draw a patient's blood, and he says that he is highly allergic to latex. How should you respond to this statement?

BIBLIOGRAPHY

Daigneault, R. (1990, January). A surprise visit from OSHA. *Medical Laboratory Observer*, pp. 31–34.

Doyle, E. T. (1991, December 16). Protecting laboratory workers. *MT Today*, pp. 1–9.

Fed. Reg. 29 C.F.R. § 1910, 1020, Vol. 56 (235) (1991).

Garner, J. S., & Simmons, B. P. (1983). *CDC guideline for isolation precautions in hospitals.* Springfield, VA: National Technical Information Service.

Moya, C. E., Guarda, L. A., & Sodeman, T. M. (1980). Safety in the clinical laboratory. Part 1: Hazard identification system and Part 2: Fire protection, prevention and control. *Laboratory Medicine, 11*(9), pp. 576–581.

National Committee for Clinical Laboratory Standards. (1991). *Protection of laboratory workers from infectious disease transmitted by blood, body fluids, and tissue* (2nd ed.). Approved Standard. NCCLS Document M29-T2. Villanova, PA: Author.

Chapter 3

PHLEBOTOMY EQUIPMENT

O B J E C T I V E S

···

After studying this chapter, you should be able to:

1. Describe the basic units of the metric system.
2. Describe the proper use of syringes in specimen collection.
3. State the relationship between bore size and the gauge of the needle.
4. Explain the principle of the evacuated system.
5. State the manner in which the following anticoagulants prevent coagulation: fluoride/oxalate, citrates, EDTA, and heparin.
6. Name the anticoagulant associated with the following color-coded tubes: blue, gray, green, and lavender.
7. State the anticoagulant that requires a 1:9 ratio of anticoagulant to blood.
8. State the purpose of the following additives: silicon coating, silica particles, and thixotropic gel.
9. Describe the three basic types of tourniquets.
10. Explain how a tourniquet makes the veins more prominent.

11. Define *hemoconcentration*.
12. Describe the different type of lancets that may be used in skin puncture.
13. List the different types of microcollection equipment available.

KEY TERMS

Additive	Any material placed in a tube that maintains or facilitates the integrity and function of the specimen.
Capillary Action	Adhesive molecular forces between liquid and solid materials that draw liquid into a narrow bore capillary tube.
Diluent	Substance used to dilute a product.
Flea	Metal rod used for mixing the blood sample that fits inside a capillary tube.
Hemostasis	The process of the formation of a blood clot when an injury occurs and then lysing of that blood clot when the injury has been repaired.
Palpate	To search for a vein with a pressure and release touch.
Reagent	Substance used to detect or measure another substance.
Thixotropic Separator Gel	A gel material capable of forming an interface between the cells and fluid portion of the blood as a result of centrifugation.
Tourniquet	Any constrictor used to facilitate vein prominence.
Vasoconstriction	The constriction of vessel(s) that limits the blood flow.

THE METRIC SYSTEM

Before a discussion of phlebotomy equipment can begin, a review of the metric system is essential. The metric system is a group of units used to make measurements, such as length, volume, temperature, weight, and time. To function in the health care setting, a knowledge of the metric system is necessary. Most metric units have a prefix that tells the relationship of that unit to the basic unit. These prefixes are the same throughout the metric system and help to simplify it. Latin prefixes show divisions of the basic units. For example, *centi* means one-hundredth and *milli* means one-thousandth of the basic unit. Greek prefixes show multiples of the basic unit. For example, *hecto* means 100 times, *kilo* means 1,000 times, and *mega* means 1,000,000 times.

The meter (M) is the basis unit for measuring length. A meter is slightly longer than a yard. Short lengths are measured as centimeters (cm) or millimeters (mm). A physician describing the length of a person's finger describes it in terms of centimeters. If the physician was describing a tumor the size of a pea, he would describe it in terms of millimeters.

Volume measurements tell the size of a box in terms of cubic units. For example, a box 1 meter tall, 1 meter wide, and 1 meter deep has a volume of 1 cubic meter. A box measuring 1 centimeter square has a volume of 1 cubic centimeter (cc). The volume of a liquid is measured in terms of liters (L). Soft drinks often come in 1- or 2-liter bottles. One-tenth of a liter is a deciliter (dl). One-thousandth of a liter is a milliliter (ml). Liquids also can take up volume. One milliliter of liquid occupies the same volume as 1 cubic centimeter. One milliliter equals 1 cubic centimeter. A 10-milliliter (10-ml) syringe is the same size as a 10-cubic centimeter (10-cc) syringe. Often in conversation, the terms *cubic centimeter* and *milliliter* are used interchangeably.

The metric system measures temperature in degrees Celsius (°C). Water freezes at 0° Celsius and boils at 100° Celsius. The normal human body temperature is 37° Celsius.

A kilogram is the basic unit of weight in the metric system. One kilogram equals 2.2046 pounds. A gram is for smaller weight and equals one-thousandth of a kilogram.

Time in the metric system, like all other systems, uses hours, minutes, and seconds. Much of the health care system uses 24-hour clock time (military time). Rather than A.M. and P.M., the clock goes a full 24 hours. For example, noon is 1200, 4 P.M. is 1600, 6 P.M. is 1800, and midnight is 2400.

SYRINGES AND NEEDLES

All methods of venipuncture require the invasive procedure of entering a vein to obtain a blood sample. The syringe and needle method is one of the oldest methods known that does not destroy

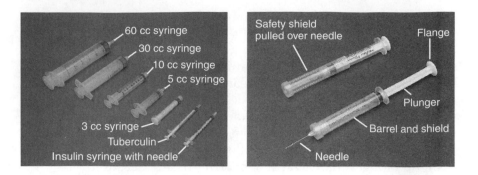

Figure 3.1 *(A) Various sizes of disposable syringes. Note size difference of tuberculin and insulin syringes. (B) A type of safety syringe. Note. From* Comprehensive Medical Assisting, Administrative and Clinical Competencies *(p. 643), by W. Lindh, M. S. Pooler, D. C. Tamparo, and J. U. Cerrato, 1998, Albany, NY: Delmar Publishers. Copyright 1998 by Delmar Publishers. Reprinted with permission.*

the integrity of the vein. Apparatus similar to the syringe and needle systems of today have been found in Egyptian tombs. The purpose of the system then was probably not to draw blood but was possibly a pus extractor or a miniature flame thrower. The principle and basic construction of the system have remained the same: a sleeve with a plunger that fits inside, and a needle attached to the other end. Syringes are now made of either glass or plastic, with the majority plastic. The barrel and plunger (Figure 3.1) varies in volume from 1 ml up to 60 ml. The barrel of the syringe is graduated into milliliters. Pulling on the plunger creates a vacuum within the barrel. The plunger on a syringe often sticks and is hard to pull. A technique called *breathing the syringe* needs to be done before it is used. To breathe the syringe, pull back on the plunger to about halfway up the barrel and then push the plunger back. This makes the plunger pull more smoothly and not have the tendency to jerk when first pulled. A jerking action while drawing blood both hurts the patient and possibly prevents the phlebotomist from obtaining an adequate blood sample.

The vacuum created by pulling on the plunger while a needle is in a patient's vein fills the syringe with blood. The larger the syringe, the greater the amount of vacuum obtained. Too large a vacuum has the tendency to pull too hard on the vein and collapse the vein. Pulling the plunger slowly and resting between pulls allows the vein time to refill with blood and prevents collapse of the vein. Generally syringes are used for the difficult-to-draw patients who have fragile, thin, or "rolly" veins that tend to

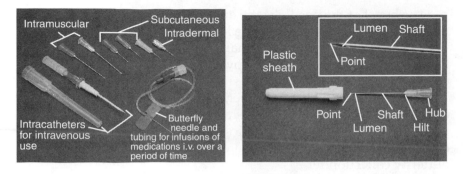

Figure 3.2 *(A) Various sizes and types of disposable needles. (B) parts of a needle and needle sheath. Note. From* Comprehensive Medical Assisting, Administrative and Clinical Competencies *(p. 644), by W. Lindh, M. S. Pooler, D. C. Tamparo, and J. U. Cerrato, 1998, Albany, NY: Delmar Publishers. Copyright 1998 by Delmar Publishers. Reprinted with permission.*

collapse when using an evacuated system. Pediatric or geriatric patients typically have these veins. The surface veins on the feet or back of the hands may also require the syringe technique. The use of a syringe and needle is limited by the capacity of the syringe. The use of a syringe larger than 10–15 ml is not recommended. If a large amount of blood is needed, a butterfly collection set should be used. This device is discussed later in the chapter. Syringes are also used in special procedures when the blood must be drawn and then transferred to a different container.

The needle used on the syringe consists of a hub, cannula (shaft), and bevel (Figure 3.2). The hub of the needle attaches to the syringe. The needle is attached by sliding the hub onto the syringe or by screwing the hub into a threaded insert called a Luer lock. The recommended length of the needle is 1 inch to 1 1/2 inches in length. The gauge of the needle is the bore size of the hole in the needle. The gauges of needles used in health care are 25, 23, 22, 21, 20, 18, 16 (from smallest to largest). The 22-, 21-, and 20-gauge needles are used for venipuncture. The 22-gauge needle is used for small veins or for pediatric patients. Use of a smaller needle may destroy red blood cells as they are pulled through the needle bore. A 23-gauge needle can be used in combination with a butterfly collection set. A 25-gauge needle cannot be used for venipuncture, because the red blood cells would be destroyed when the blood is pulled through the bore of the needle. The 25-gauge needle is used for intermuscular injections. The 18- and 16-gauge needles are used for the infusion of fluids or blood products or the removal of blood during the donor process.

The bevel of the needle is the angle the needle has been cut on the tip. The sharper the bevel, the less pain the needle produces. The length of the bevel must remain small enough to fit within the lumen of the vein. Needles are now manufactured with laser-cut bevels for smooth edges and are silicon coated for easy insertion. The walls of the needle are thinner, so it has a thinner outside diameter and therefore makes a smaller hole as it enters the patient's arm. These characteristics of a syringe needle are duplicated in the needles of the evacuated tube system and the butterfly collection set.

EVACUATED SYSTEM

The evacuated system is often called the Vacutainer system. Vacutainer can be a misnomer because the term *Vacutainer* is a brand name for the evacuated system manufactured by the Becton Dickinson Company. Phlebotomists will often say Vacutainer when they are using another company's product. This is the same as saying you are eating Jell-O when actually you are eating a generic brand of gelatin. The evacuated tube system has been manufactured since the 1940s.

The evacuated blood collection system uses the principle that a syringe creates a vacuum when the plunger is pulled. In the evacuated system, a tube with a vacuum already in it attaches to the needle and the tube's vacuum is replaced by blood. The system consists of a double-pointed needle, a plastic holder, and a series of vacuum tubes with rubber stoppers (Figure 3.3).

The reason the system works so well is because of the needle. The needle is double-pointed with a needle on each end and a screw hub near the center. The needle extending from the holder has the proper bevel to pierce the skin and enter the vein. The needle within the holder pierces the rubber stopper on the evacuated tube. This needle has a rubber sleeve that covers it (Figure 3.4). The sleeve works as a valve that stops the flow of blood when the tube is removed. Pushing the tube into the holder compresses the rubber sleeve and exposes the needle, allowing it to enter the tube. When the tube is being removed, the sleeve slides back over the needle and stops the flow of blood. The needle entering the patient varies in length from 1 inch to 1 1/2 inches. The gauges available are 20, 21, and 22. The 21 and 22 gauges are the most common. The gauge refers to the size of the bore in the needle shaft, also known as the lumen of the needle. One of the most recent improvements has been to manufacture

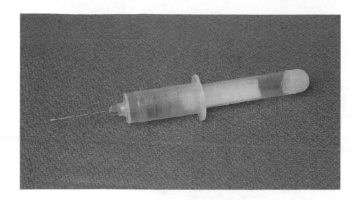

Figure 3.3 *Evacuated blood collection system. Note. From* Comprehensive Medical Assisting, Administrative and Clinical Competencies *(p. 826), by W. Lindh, M. S. Pooler, D. C. Tamparo, and J. U. Cerrato, 1998, Albany, NY: Delmar Publishers. Copyright 1998 by Delmar Publishers. Reprinted with permission.*

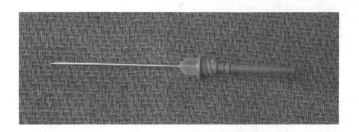

Figure 3.4 *Evacuated blood collection system needle. Note. From* Comprehensive Medical Assisting, Administrative and Clinical Competencies *(p. 826), by W. Lindh, M. S. Pooler, D. C. Tamparo, and J. U. Cerrato, 1998, Albany, NY: Delmar Publishers. Copyright 1998 by Delmar Publishers. Reprinted with permission.*

needles with a thinner wall. With a thinner wall, the needle still draws at a normal rate, but it hurts less because the needle has a smaller outside diameter. Silicon coats the needles so they slide into the skin with less resistance. The needle can be thought of as a pipeline that delivers blood from the patient to the tube. The tube is the method by which the blood is pumped from the patient. The blood fills the tube because of the vacuum of the tube.

The bevel of the needle is the slanted opening at the end of the needle. It must always be facing upward when the needle is inserted into the vein. When you look straight down on the needle as the needle is inserted into the skin, the opening in the needle should be visible. The bevel of the needle is cut at an angle so that when the needle is inserted into the skin the bevel angle ensures

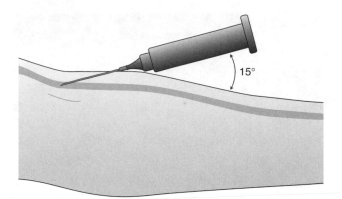

Figure 3.5 *Proper angle of needle insertion for venipuncture. Note. From* Comprehensive Medical Assisting, Administrative and Clinical Competencies *(p. 826), by W. Lindh, M. S. Pooler, D. C. Tamparo, and J. U. Cerrato, 1998, Albany, NY: Delmar Publishers. Copyright 1998 by Delmar Publishers. Reprinted with permission.*

maximum blood flow through the needle. To obtain this maximum blood flow, the needle should be inserted at a 15-degree angle to the surface of the skin (Figure 3.5).

The holder for the needle makes the task of collecting the blood sample easier. It gives the phlebotomist something more substantial to hold on to and a way to center the needle into the stopper of the evacuated tube. The needle screws into the holder, and the tube inserts into the other end of the holder. The holder has an indentation about 1/4 inch from the hub of the needle. This indentation marks the point where the short end of the needle starts to enter the rubber stopper of the tube. If the tube is inserted past this point before you have entered the vein, the tube will fill with air and not produce a blood sample. To do a venipuncture, grasp the holder the same way as you would hold the barrel of a syringe. The holders come in two sizes: one size for adult venipuncture and one size for small-diameter tubes used in pediatrics. The holders have been under a constant state of change to reduce needlestick injuries. The holders have changed from the basic style (Figure 3.6) to styles that cover the needle after use (Figure 3.7). These styles vary from holders that slide an outer sleeve over the contaminated needle to a holder that snaps a cover over the needle. These styles require that the entire holder and needle be discarded after use.

A variation on this is the Bio-Plexus Puncture-Guard needle, which has a blunting cannula that covers the needlepoint when the phlebotomist applies pressure to the blood collection tube

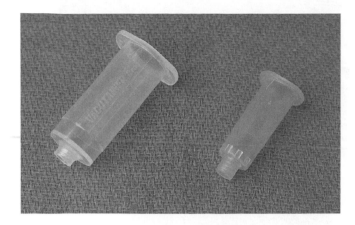

Figure 3.6 *Evacuated tube system holders: (A) adult holder, (B) pediatric holder. Note.* From Comprehensive Medical Assisting, Administrative and Clinical Competencies *(p. 826), by W. Lindh, M. S. Pooler, D. C. Tamparo, and J. U. Cerrato, 1998, Albany, NY: Delmar Publishers. Copyright 1998 by Delmar Publishers. Reprinted with permission.*

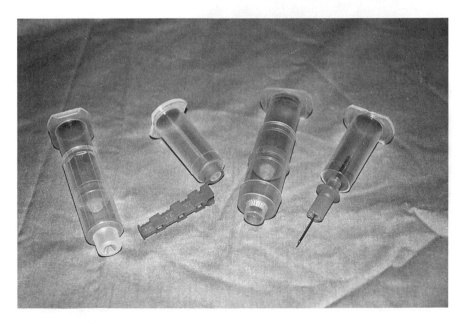

Figure 3.7 *Safety-evacuated tube system holders; discard after use.*

(Figure 3.8). Blunting the needle before it is removed from the patient virtually eliminates the potential for needlestick.

An alternative to sliding a sleeve over the needle is to have a quick release of the needle from the holder. Alternate styles of needle holders permit the user to remove the needle and use the

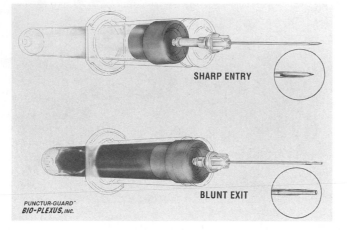

Figure 3.8 *The Bio-Plexis Puncture Guard self-blunting blood collection needle and vacuum tube system with self blunt-end cannula within needle. (Illustration courtesy of Bio-Plexis, Inc., Tolland, CT.)*

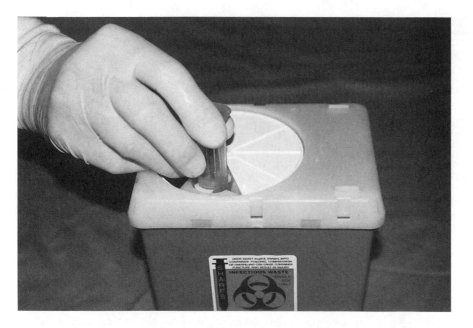

Figure 3.9 *Sharps container and needle holder that when combined offer a quick, one-handed needle release.*

holder again. Several variations in design are available. Figure 3.9 shows a sharps container and needle holder that when combined offer a quick one-handed needle release. The Vacutainer brand Pronto Quick Release Needle Holder (Figure 3.10) has a quick-release button to release the needle without the need for a specific

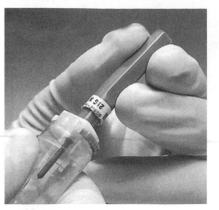

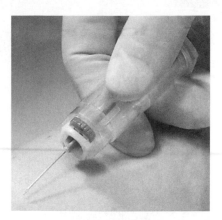

1. Thread needle. Note: if the needle is threaded too tightly, the over torque mechanism will automatically open.

2. Perform venipuncture.

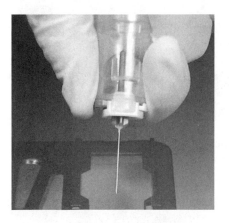

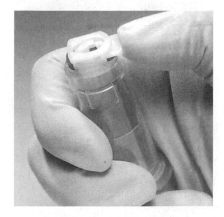

3. In downward position, place needle over opening of sharps container, push green release button.

4. To reuse, push white reset button.

Figure 3.10 *Vacutainer brand Pronto Quick Release Needle Holder. (Courtesy of Becton Dickinson Vacutainer Systems.)*

sharps container. These do not eliminate the potential for needle-stick between the venipuncture and final disposal but allow the user to reuse the holder and reduce the cost.

The Vacutainer brand Safety-Gard Phlebotomy System combines the benefits of the sleeve sliding over the needle at the point of use and the quick release of the needle (Figure 3.11). This

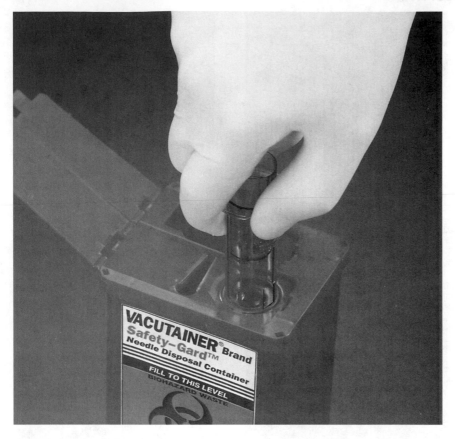

- User retracts needle into holder at point of use
- Container permits one-handed disposal of enclosed needle

Figure 3.11   *Vacutainer brand Safety-Gard Phlebotomy System. (Courtesy of Becton Dickinson Vacutainer Systems.)*

system requires a paired needle holder and sharps container for effective use.

Evacuated collection tubes contain a vacuum with a rubber stopper sealing the tube. These tubes range in size from 2.0 ml to 15 ml. The tubes are sterile or nonsterile, but most of the tubes used now are sterile to prevent contamination of the specimen and the patient. The patient can obtain an infection from a nonsterile tube if the blood flows into the tube, becomes contaminated, and then backflows into the patient. The patient will then be injected with the contaminating organism and possibly develop an infection. A sterile tube does not contaminate the blood, so any backflow of blood is inconsequential.

The tubes are glass or plastic and vary in length from 65 mm to 127 mm with an external diameter of 10 mm, 13 mm, or 16 mm.

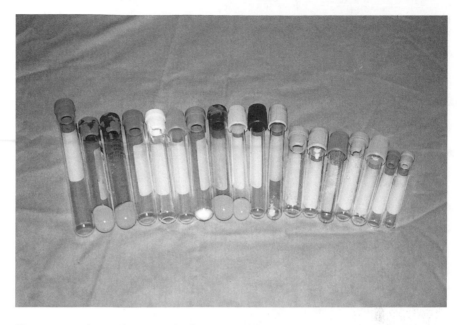

Figure 3.12 *Assorted evacuated tubes.*

The diameter is such that it will easily slide into the evacuated system holder. The 10-mm size fits perfectly into the pediatric holder; the 13- and 16-mm sizes slide easily into the adult holder (Figure 3.12). The mechanism of the rubber stopper on the tube has changed because of the increase of blood and body fluid precautions. The traditional rubber stopper popped as the top was removed to access the specimen. This created an aerosol that could be inhaled or ingested. Becton Dickinson developed a tube called Hemogard (Figure 3.13). This tube has a plastic sleeve that fits over the rubber stopper to contain any aerosols that might be dispersed when the cap is removed. The Hemogard cap has no benefits for the phlebotomist but is an excellent safeguard for the technologist working with the sample.

Tubes have an expiration date on each tube to indicate when the tube should no longer be used. The tubes are good until the end of the month stamped on the tube. After the expiration date, the vacuum will possibly not fill the tube completely and the additives are not guaranteed to perform as designed. Using tubes past the expiration date compromises the integrity of the specimen and can give questionable results.

Tubes made from plastic are now used more frequently in health care settings. Only recently have plastics been developed that can maintain a vacuum within the tube. Plastic is permeable,

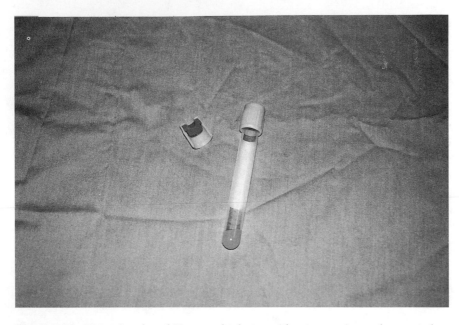

Figure 3.13   *Vacutainer brand Hemogard tube top with cutaway view and evacuated tube. (Courtesy Becton Dickinson Vacutainer Systems.)*

and the vacuum used to leak out in a short period of time. Plastic tubes are manufactured with or without anticoagulant.

Various additives are added to the tubes to improve the quality of the specimen. These **additives** are not anticoagulants or preservatives but are used to improve specimen quality or to accelerate specimen processing. Most tubes have a silicon coating on the interior surface. This silicon fills the microscopically rough surface of the glass. Glass may feel smooth to the touch, but it has a rough surface that cells can stick to. The silicon fills in these cracks and crevasses and prevents the cells from adhering to the glass surface. This reduces the chance for hemolysis and makes the sides slicker so the cells can centrifuge to the bottom of the tube faster. These tubes have a red stopper, red/black stopper, or gold stopper (Hemogard tube) depending on the manufacturer. Some serum tubes have a clot activator that speeds the clotting process. This clot activator consists of silica particles on the sides of the tubes that initiate the clotting process.

A type of clot activator that is used for stat (emergency) testing is thrombin. The thrombin is within the tube to hasten the clotting process faster than the silica particles.

Serum and plasma tubes can also be purchased with a **thixotrophic separator gel** (Figure 3.14). This gel is an inert

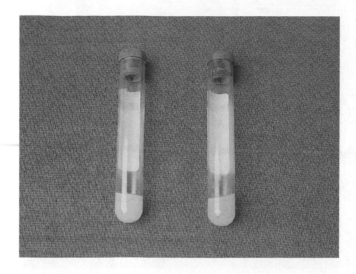

Figure 3.14 *Thixotrophic separator gel tubes. Note. From* Comprehensive Medical Assisting, Administrative and Clinical Competencies *(p. 828), by W. Lindh, M. S. Pooler, D. C. Tamparo, and J. U. Cerrato, 1998, Albany, NY: Delmar Publishers. Copyright 1998 by Delmar Publishers. Reprinted with permission.*

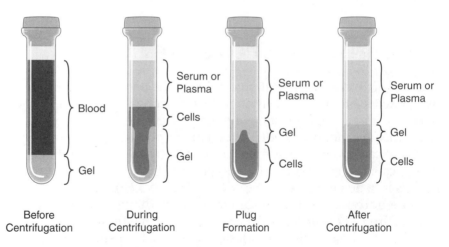

Figure 3.15 *Separator gel tube: centrifugation process. Note. From* Comprehensive Medical Assisting, Administrative and Clinical Competencies *(p. 828), by W. Lindh, M. S. Pooler, D. C. Tamparo, and J. U. Cerrato, 1998, Albany, NY: Delmar Publishers. Copyright 1998 by Delmar Publishers. Reprinted with permission.*

material that undergoes a temporary change in viscosity during centrifugation. It has a density that is intermediate to cells/clot and plasma/serum. When centrifuged, the gel moves up the sides of the tube and engulfs the cells/clot, and an interface of gel forms that separates the cells/clot from the plasma/serum (Figure 3.15).

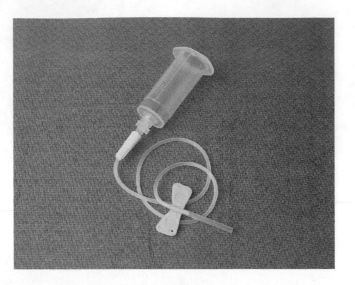

Figure 3.16 *Butterfly collection set/winged infusion set. Note. From* Comprehensive Medical Assisting, Administrative and Clinical Competencies *(p. 839), by W. Lindh, M. S. Pooler, D. C. Tamparo, and J. U. Cerrato, 1998, Albany, NY: Delmar Publishers. Copyright 1998 by Delmar Publishers. Reprinted with permission.*

BUTTERFLY COLLECTION SYSTEM

The butterfly collection system combines the benefits of the evacuated system and the syringe system. It has a 21- or 23-gauge needle with attached plastic wings on one end. A 3- to 12-inch tubing leads from the needle. On the other end of this tubing is a hub that can attach to a syringe. A needle covered by a rubber sleeve can also be attached to this tubing. This covered needle screws into an evacuated tube holder (Figure 3.16).

The butterfly system is for small veins that are difficult to draw with the other systems. Holding the plastic wings attached to the needle provides easy access into small surface veins on the back of the hand, the arm, or the foot. Instead of entering the vein at the usual 15-degree angle, the winged needle is inserted at approximately a 5-degree angle and then threaded into the vein. This procedure anchors the needle in the center of even a small vein. If the patient moves, the tubing is flexible so the needle stays anchored and does not pull out of the vein. The butterfly collection set works well on children who have both small veins and the tendency to move while blood is being collected. The tubing also works as a pressure relief valve. A large evacuated tube or large syringe can be attached to the tubing, and the vein will not collapse as would normally occur.

The system also offers the flexibility to start drawing blood with a syringe and then finish with the evacuated tube system. A syringe can be drawn for procedures that require a syringe sample, and then the syringe can be removed and the evacuated tube system attached for multiple tube collection. Even with all of these benefits, the butterfly collection set is not used for all collection. It is much more expensive than the needle system. This additional expense is not justified for the majority of venipunctures.

COAGULATION

Before an explanation of anticoagulants can begin, the process of coagulation must be explained. A simple example was given in Figure 1.12. **Hemostasis** is a coagulation process causing the formation of a blood clot when an injury occurs and then lysing of that blood clot when the injury has been repaired.

Primary hemostasis is the first step of the process. In this primary phase, the damaged vessel(s) constrict to limit the blood flow to the injury. This **vasoconstriction** limits bleeding from the injury. Then the platelets clump to form a temporary plug by sticking to one another in a process called platelet aggregation. This is all that is needed to heal some injuries such as a needle puncture of a vein. Primary hemostasis has traditionally been tested for by the bleeding time test (discussed in Chapter 6). Newer methods now test the platelet function by using a blood sample rather than a time-dependent skin cut.

Secondary hemostasis is needed for more serious injuries and involves the formation of a fibrin clot. This involves a complex series of interactions in which one factor activates the next factor in a coagulation cascade. The factors are designated by Roman numerals. The coagulation cascade is divided into two separate intrinsic and extrinsic pathways that come together to form a common pathway (Figure 3.17). The intrinsic pathway begins with Factor XII and is measured by the activated partial thromboplastin time (APTT) test. The APTT test is also used to monitor heparin therapy of an individual. The extrinsic pathway begins with Factor VII and is measured by the prothrombin time (PT) test. The PT test is also used to monitor warfarin therapy.

In the common pathway, prothrombin is converted to thrombin, and fibrinogen then converts into fibrin to form a fibrin plug, which is also known as the hemostatic plug. Once the injury

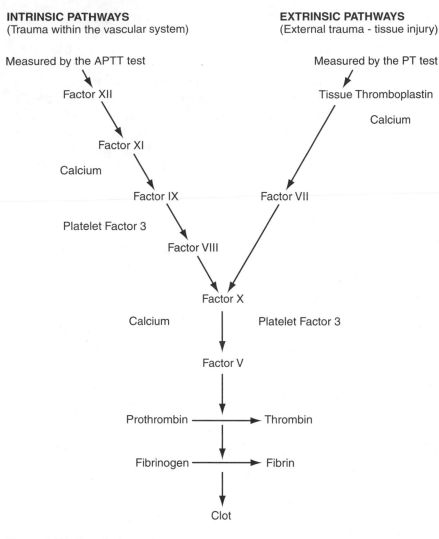

INTRINSIC PATHWAYS
(Trauma within the vascular system)

EXTRINSIC PATHWAYS
(External trauma - tissue injury)

Measured by the APTT test

Measured by the PT test

Factor XII

Tissue Thromboplastin

Calcium

Factor XI

Calcium

Factor IX   Factor VII

Platelet Factor 3

Factor VIII

Factor X

Calcium   Platelet Factor 3

Factor V

Prothrombin ——————▶ Thrombin

Fibrinogen ——————▶ Fibrin

Clot

Figure 3.17 *Coagulation pathways.*

is repaired, fibrinolysis occurs to break down the fibrin clot into small fragments called fibrin degradation products (FDPs).

This coagulation cascade is simplified in Figure 3.18. The blood tubes that contain an anticoagulant prevent the coagulation cascade from going to completion in the tube. If the required specimen is a serum sample, then the tube that is used will allow the blood to clot and the coagulation cascade is completed.

This coagulation cascade is important in preventing blood from clotting in the tubes that are collected. Some tests require a

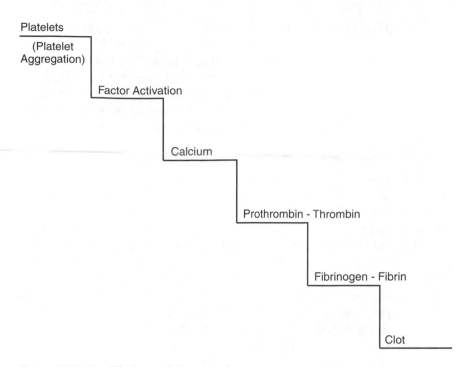

Figure 3.18 *Simplified coagulation cascade.*

whole blood or plasma specimen and need to be drawn in a specimen tube that is not allowed to clot. To prevent the blood from clotting, the tube contains a chemical anticoagulant. This anticoagulant works by stopping the clotting process by removing the calcium through the formation of calcium salts or by inhibiting the conversion of prothrombin to thrombin.

Both calcium and thrombin are part of the coagulation cascade. The coagulation cascade is like a staircase in which a ball is bounced down each step. The blood clots when the ball reaches the bottom of the stairs. If a step is taken away, the ball does not reach the bottom of the stairs and the blood does not clot. This staircase contains many steps. These steps consist of different chemicals and factors that are required for a person's blood to clot. A person with a bleeding disorder will have one of the factors missing or will be physically unable to use a needed chemical. One patient of this type is a hemophiliac. The patient can temporarily overcome this bleeding disorder by receiving an appropriate factor. The hemophiliac has one of the steps in the staircase missing. By giving the hemophiliac a factor such as Factor VIII, the step is rebuilt and clotting occurs.

ANTICOAGULANTS

Clotting can be stopped in the test tube. A tube that has an antico-agulant removes one of the steps to the staircase, and the blood does not clot. The anticoagulant prevents clotting depending on the anticoagulant used. The common anticoagulants used consist of fluoride/oxalates, citrates, ethylenediaminetetraacetic acid (EDTA), or heparin.

Gray-stoppered tubes contain oxalates in combination with another weak anticoagulant, sodium fluoride. The anticoagulant combination of potassium oxalate and sodium fluoride works by precipitating out the calcium in the blood and therefore stopping the coagulation cascade. The fluoride's primary function is not an anticoagulant but a glycolytic inhibitor. The fluoride preserves the glucose in the blood sample by inhibiting the enzymes involved in breakdown of the glucose (glycolysis). As a blood sample sits without the fluoride, the glucose is broken down at a rate of around 7 percent per hour. A blood sample that is drawn from a patient into a plain red-stoppered tube will have nothing in that sample to preserve it, or to keep it from clotting. As the sample sits, the glucose in the sample will be utilized by the blood cells. The glucose molecules will be broken down, and the amount of glucose in the patient's sample will decrease. The fluoride in the gray-stoppered tube prevents the glucose from being utilized by the cells.

A sample that is drawn from a patient often has a time delay before it is tested at the laboratory. What is monitored is the glucose of that patient at the time the sample was drawn. If the glucose were allowed to decrease in the sample, the results at the time of testing would indicate the patient had a glucose value less than actual. The patient could then be falsely treated for a low glucose, or a patient who was running a high value might appear as normal. The way to prevent this is to draw samples to be tested for glucose in a gray-stoppered tube if there is to be a delay in testing.

Light-blue-stoppered tubes contain the anticoagulant sodium citrate. The sodium citrate prevents the coagulation by binding calcium in a nonionized form. The sodium citrate anticoagulant is in the concentration 3.8 percent sodium citrate (0.129 M) or 3.2 percent sodium citrate (0.105 M). The correct concentration of sodium citrate must be used to have consistent results for the patient. It is critical that the light-blue tubes drawn be filled to their proper level for accurate patient results. A ratio of one part of anticoagulant to nine parts blood must be maintained. If a tube is only half filled, the ratio will be off and the results will be invalid. The anticoagulant in the tube prevents the blood from clotting by binding the calcium. To test the blood for coagulation studies, the blood is centrifuged to produce a plasma specimen. An aliquot of this plasma specimen combines with other chemicals to restart the coagulation process and produce a clot. The time it takes for a visible clot to form is the result of the coagulation study. There are normal time ranges for this clotting to occur, and an abnormal patient will fall outside these results. Three such tests using the light-blue-stoppered tube to detect clotting problems are PT, APTT, and fibrinogen assay. These tests will give prolonged results if the tube is not filled to the proper level. These prolonged results will cause the physician to reduce the patient's medication when it was the inaccurate filling of the tube that changed the patient's results.

Citrate is not only used in the light-blue-stoppered tube. It is used extensively as the anticoagulant in routine blood donor bags. The citrate is in the form of citrate-phosphate-dextrose-adenine-1 (CPDA-1). This form of citrate both prevents the blood from clotting and preserves the viability of the erythrocytes. Weeks after the blood was drawn from the donor, the erythrocytes are capable of transporting oxygen to the tissues. The anticoagulant is still in a 1:9 ratio with 63 ml of anticoagulant and approximately 450 ml of blood. Citrate is also found in a yellow-stoppered tube. This tube has as an additive a solution called ACD. This additive is either solution A or solution B. The difference in the solutions depends on the concentration of trisodium citrate, citric acid, and dextrose solution. The tube has a variety of uses in testing in blood banks with tissue typing, DNA testing, and paternity testing.

A yellow-stoppered tube that does not contain citrate is used for collecting blood culture samples. This yellow-stoppered tube looks the same as the two previous tubes except it contains the additive sodium polyethol sulfonate and sodium chloride. The yellow-stoppered tube can be confusing in that there are multiple types of yellow-stoppered tubes with specific uses. The phlebotomist must read the label before using one of these tubes to ensure that the proper tube with the proper additive is used.

The lavender tubes contain the anticoagulant EDTA. This anticoagulant also binds the calcium to prevent coagulation. This EDTA is in the form of tripotassium EDTA or dipotassium EDTA. Tripotassium EDTA is used in glass tubes and is in the liquid form. Dipotassium EDTA is in plastic tubes and is in a spray-dried powder form. Either form is the anticoagulant of choice for hematology procedures. This anticoagulant preserves the cell morphology for CBCs and differential blood smears. Other anticoagulants distort the size and shape of the cells. This distortion often mimics the appearance of a disease process when it is really the effects of the anticoagulant.

Up to this point, all the anticoagulants discussed have prevented coagulation by precipitating or binding the calcium in the blood. The green tubes contain heparin, which stops the coagulation by inhibiting the conversion of prothrombin to thrombin and thus the following stages that lead to a clot. What has occurred is that no fibrin is formed to cause a clot. Heparin is a naturally occurring substance that is present in most of our tissues, but at low levels. Thus it has the least effect of all the anticoagulants on clinical chemistry tests. It produces the least stress on erythrocytes and minimizes hemolysis. Heparin is the anticoagulant of choice for pH determinations, electrolyte studies, and arterial blood gases. Heparin comes in two forms, either lithium heparin or sodium heparin. Before drawing a test with a heparin tube, you must know what type of heparin is acceptable. Heparin is not acceptable for blood samples that may be stored for more than 48 hours before testing. After this time, heparinized blood will slowly begin to clot, forming small fibrin strands.

A royal-blue-stoppered tube is used for trace element studies. The tubes are used for analysis of such trace elements as lead, zinc, arsenic, or copper. The patient contacts these elements through occupational or environmental exposure. Normal serum or plasma blood tubes cannot be used. In the normal manufacture of the glass and rubber contained within the tubes, the trace elements are present. If blood was drawn into normal tubes, the trace elements would leach out of the glass and rubber stopper to falsely elevate the results. The trace element tubes use a specially refined glass and rubber to avoid this. The royal-blue tube comes in three varieties. One contains no anticoagulant and produces a clot specimen; the other two have sodium heparin or sodium EDTA as an anticoagulant.

All tubes that have any type of additive must be gently inverted immediately after collection. The additives do not mix with the blood as the blood enters the tube. The mixing will only be complete with eight to ten gentle inversions of the tube. The tube should never be shaken.

TOURNIQUETS

The **tourniquet** constricts the flow of blood in the arm and makes the veins more prominent. The most commonly used tourniquet is a soft, pliable rubber strip approximately 1 inch wide by 15–18

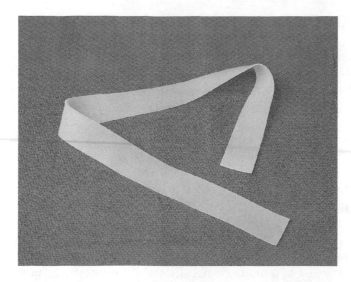

Figure 3.19 *Soft latex tourniquet. Note. From* Comprehensive Medical Assisting, Administrative and Clinical Competencies *(p. 829), by W. Lindh, M. S. Pooler, D. C. Tamparo, and J. U. Cerrato, 1998, Albany, NY: Delmar Publishers. Copyright 1998 by Delmar Publishers. Reprinted with permission.*

inches long. This rubber strip serves as a universal tourniquet for all conditions. Velcro strips are also available, and round rubber tubing is occasionally used. The rubber strip is the most widely used because it can easily be released with one hand. Being about 1 inch wide, it does not cut into the patient's arm but distributes the pressure. The tourniquet can easily be wiped off with alcohol to prevent spreading of infection and is inexpensive enough that it can be replaced often (Figure 3.19).

The tourniquet is applied 3–4 inches above the puncture site. It is applied tight enough to slow the flow of blood in the veins but not prevent the flow of blood in the arteries. The process is very similar to damming a small stream. By damming the stream, the water forms a pond in front of the dam. With the tourniquet applied, the arteries fill the veins with blood, pooling the blood in the veins before the tourniquet. This pooling of blood makes the veins more prominent. The veins can then be **palpated** to determine their direction, depth, and size. The tourniquet should be on the arm no longer than one minute. A stream will become stagnant when it no longer flows. A tourniquet that is left on too long will cause a hemoconcentration of the blood and an increased concentration of constituents in the blood sample.

MICROCOLLECTION EQUIPMENT

Blood collections sometimes require collection by skin puncture. For this type of collection, special microcollection equipment is needed. This equipment varies in how it is used but always makes either a puncture or a cut into the skin and through the capillary bed. The equipment used to collect the blood depends on the test being performed. The equipment consists of two parts: a method of puncturing the finger and a method to collect the sample.

A number of different skin puncture lancets are commercially available to puncture the skin for an adequate blood flow. Surgical blades used in the past carried the hazard of puncturing too deeply, especially in the newborn heelstick or the pediatric patient. Lancets have now been designed for controlled depth of puncture, and surgical blades should be used only for surgery. Lancets consist of a blade or needle the phlebotomist manually punctures the skin with or a spring-loaded device that makes the puncture when the trigger is released. The hand-held lancets (Figure 3.20) are still used but have several disadvantages. The phlebotomist can limit the depth of puncture by not puncturing to the stop point on the lancet. The tendency is to be sympathetic with the patient and not stick hard enough. If this occurs,

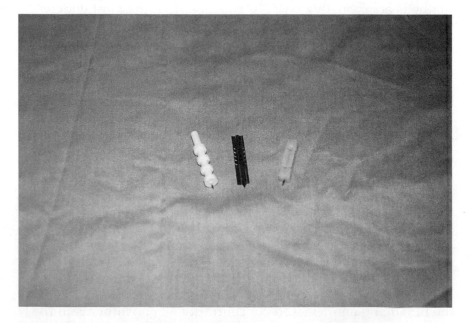

Figure 3.20 *Lancets used for manual puncture.*

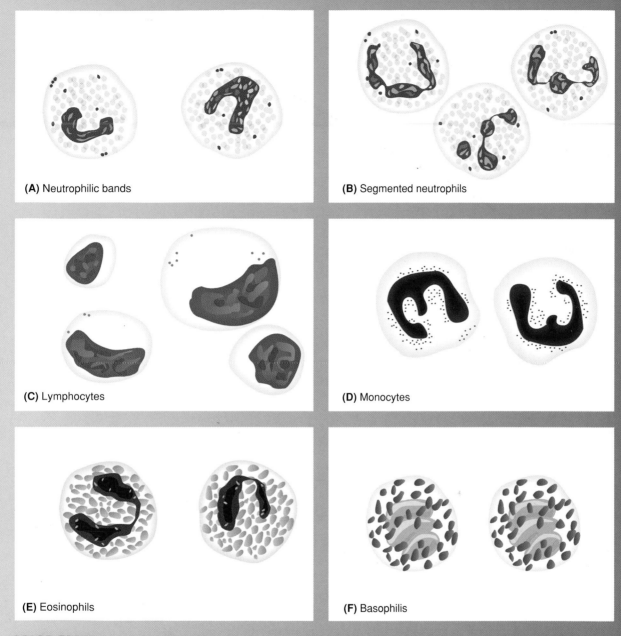

(A) Neutrophilic bands

(B) Segmented neutrophils

(C) Lymphocytes

(D) Monocytes

(E) Eosinophils

(F) Basophilis

COLOR PLATE 1 Various divisions of leukocytes from a stained blood smear.

Tube Guide

VACUTAINER BRAND TUBES WITH HEMOGARD™ CLOSURE

VACUTAINER® Tubes with HEMOGARD Closure	VACUTAINER Tubes	Additive	Number of Inversions at Blood Collection (Invert gently, do not shake)	Laboratory Use	Use these two columns for your lab's information	
					Volume Draw (ml.)	Remarks
Gold		• Clot activator and gel for serum separation	5	SST Brand Tube for serum determinations in chemistry. Tube inversions ensure mixing of clot activator with blood and clotting within 30 minutes.		
Light Green		• Lithium heparin and gel for plasma separation	8	PST Brand Tube for plasma determinations in chemistry. Tube inversions prevent clotting.		
Red		• None	0	For serum determinations in chemistry, serology and blood banking.		
Orange		• Thrombin	8	For stat serum determinations in chemistry. Tube inversions ensure complete clotting, usually in less than 5 minutes.		
Royal Blue		• Sodium heparin • Na₂EDTA • None	8 8 0	For trace element, toxicology and nutrient determinations. Special stopper formulation offers low levels of trace elements (see package insert).		
Green		• Sodium heparin • Lithium heparin • Ammonium heparin	8 8 8	For plasma determinations in chemistry. Tube inversions prevent clotting.		
Gray		• Potassium oxalate/ sodium fluoride • Sodium fluoride • Lithium iodoacetate • Lithium iodoacetate/ lithium heparin	8 8 8 8	For glucose determinations. Tube inversions ensure proper mixing of additive and blood. Oxalate and heparin, anticoagulants, will give plasma samples. Without them, samples are serum.		

COLOR PLATE 2 Tube Guide for Vacutainer Brand tubes with hemogard closure. (Courtesy of Becton Dickinson Vacutainer Systems.)

Color	Additive	Inversions	Laboratory Use
Brown	• Sodium heparin	8	For lead determinations. This tube is certified to contain less than .01 μg/mL (ppm) lead. Tube inversions prevent clotting.
Yellow	• Sodium polyanetholesulfonate (SPS)	8	For blood culture specimen collections in microbiology. Tube inversions prevent clotting.
	OR		
	• ACD - Acid Citrate Dextrose Additions: Solution A - 22.0g/L trisodium citrate, 8.0g/L citric acid, 24.5g/L dextrose Solution B - 13.2g/L trisodium citrate, 4.8g/L citric acid, 14.7g/L dextrose	8	For use in blood bank studies; HLA phenotyping, DNA and Paternity testing.
Lavender	• Liquid K_3EDTA	8	For whole blood hematology determinations. Tube inversions prevent clotting.
	• Spray-dried K_2EDTA	8	
Light Blue	• .105M sodium citrate (3.2%)	8	For coagulation determinations on plasma specimens. Tube inversions prevent clotting. NOTE: Certain tests require chilled specimens. Follow recommended procedures for collection and transport of specimen.
	• .129M sodium citrate (3.8%)	8	

Small-volume Tubes (2ml and 3ml: 13 x 75 mm)
Small-volume Tubes (2ml: 10.25 x 47 mm, 3ml: 10.25 x 64 mm)

Color	Additive	Inversions	Laboratory Use
Red	• None	0	For serum determinations in chemistry, serology and blood banking
Green	• Sodium heparin	8	For plasma determinations in chemistry. Tube inversions prevent clotting.
	• Lithium heparin	8	
Lavender	• Liquid K_3EDTA	8	For whole blood hematology determinations. Tube inversions prevent clotting.
	• Spray-dried K_2EDTA	8	
Light Blue	• .105M sodium citrate (3.2%)	8	For coagulation determinations on plasma specimens. Tube inversions prevent clotting. NOTE: Certain tests require chilled specimens. Follow recommended procedures for collection and transport of specimen.
	• .129M sodium citrate (3.8%)	8	

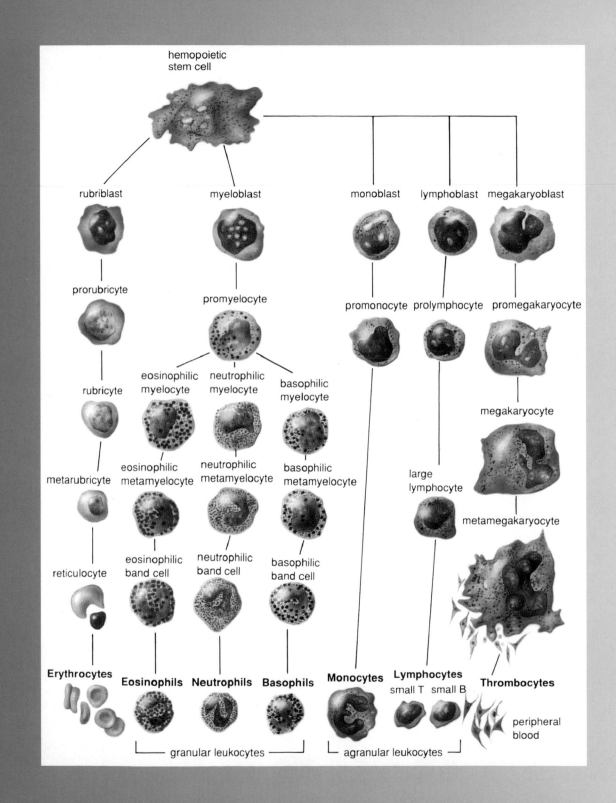

COLOR PLATE 3 Hemopoiesis showing blood cells and platelet formation starting with hemopoietic stem cell.

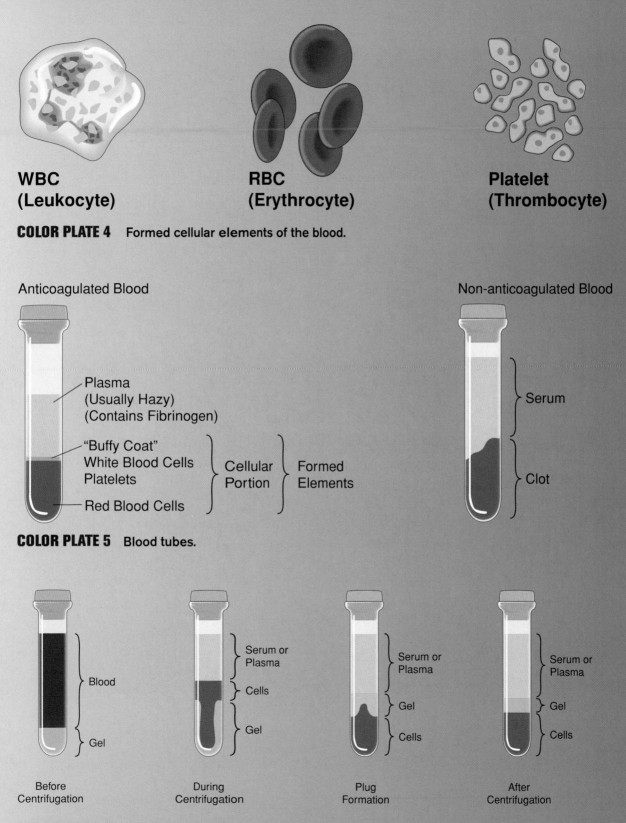

WBC
(Leukocyte)

RBC
(Erythrocyte)

Platelet
(Thrombocyte)

COLOR PLATE 4   Formed cellular elements of the blood.

Anticoagulated Blood

Non-anticoagulated Blood

Plasma
(Usually Hazy)
(Contains Fibrinogen)

"Buffy Coat"
White Blood Cells
Platelets

Red Blood Cells

Cellular
Portion

Formed
Elements

Serum

Clot

COLOR PLATE 5   Blood tubes.

Blood

Gel

Serum or
Plasma

Cells

Gel

Serum or
Plasma

Gel

Cells

Serum or
Plasma

Gel

Cells

Before
Centrifugation

During
Centrifugation

Plug
Formation

After
Centrifugation

COLOR PLATE 6   Separator gel tube: centrifugation process.

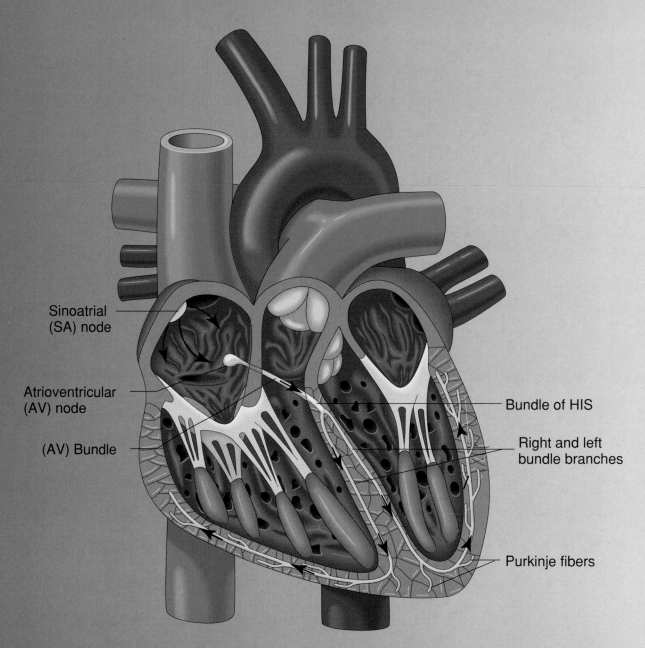

Sinoatrial (SA) node

Atrioventricular (AV) node

(AV) Bundle

Bundle of HIS

Right and left bundle branches

Purkinje fibers

COLOR PLATE 7 Conduction system of the heart.

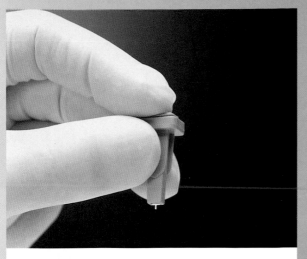

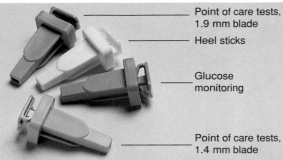

Point of care tests, 1.9 mm blade

Heel sticks

Glucose monitoring

Point of care tests, 1.4 mm blade

COLOR PLATE 8 (left)   MICROTAINER Brand lancets are available in different types for various purposes. To use, hold lancet on skin, and depress plunger with index finger to make puncture. Immediately release plunger while holding lancet on site. Discard lancet after use in biohazard container. (Courtesy of Becton Dickinson Vacutainer Systems.)

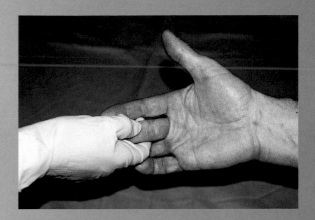

COLOR PLATE 9 (above)   Fingerstick skin puncture. (1) When the patient is in position, gently massage the entire length of the finger using a milking action. This increases the temperature of the finger and improves perfusion.

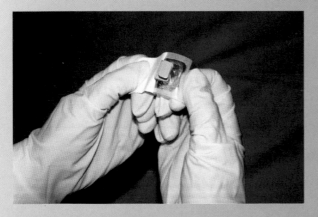

COLOR PLATE 10   Fingerstick skin puncture. (2) Clean the incision site, and let it air dry. Remove the lancet from its plastic packet, taking care not to touch or contaminate the blade slot surface.

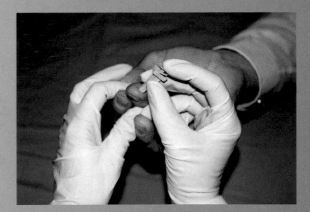

COLOR PLATE 11   Fingerstick skin puncture. (3) Massage the lower portion of the finger while avoiding the fingertip incision site. Then firmly grasp the lower portion of the finger to restrict return circulation. Firmly position the lancet device on the finger in a position to cut across the fingerprint lines. Depress the plunger with your index finger to make the puncture. Immediately release the plunger while holding the lancet on the site.

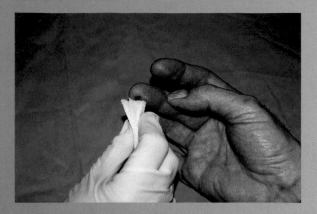

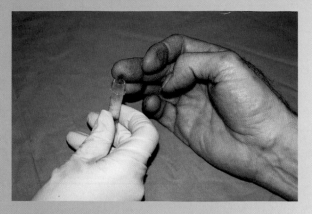

COLOR PLATE 12 After puncturing the finger, remove the lancet from the patient's finger. Using a gauze pad, gently wipe away the first droplet of blood. Gentle, continuous pressure on the finger ensures a free flow of blood.

COLOR PLATE 13 Taking care not to make direct contact between the incision and the collection container, fill to the desired volume. Following collection, gently press a dry gauze pad to the incision.

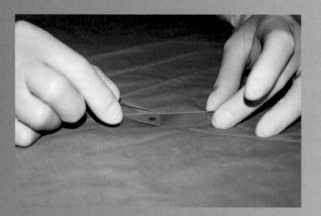

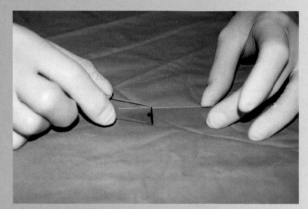

COLOR PLATE 14 Blood smear preparation. (1) Rest the end of the spreader slide at a 45-degree angle just in front of the drop of blood.

COLOR PLATE 15 Blood smear preparation. (2) Draw the spreader slide backward until it just touches the drop of blood.

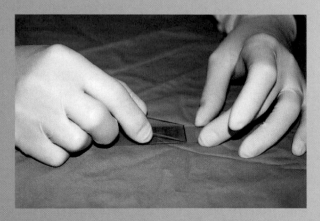

COLOR PLATE 16 Blood smear preparation. (3) Push the spreader slide rapidly across the stationary slide with an even stroke and pressure.

adequate blood flow is not obtained, and the patient has to be punctured again. Another disadvantage is that the patient can see the blade coming and becomes more apprehensive to the stick. Children can become so apprehensive that they can pull their hand out of the phlebotomist's grasp just as the phlebotomist is ready to stick. In a case like this, the phlebotomist possibly can stick himself or herself. The correct technique to puncture the patient is to block the view of the lancet so the patient will not be as apprehensive to the stick. The patient will not see the blade and will then not jerk away during the puncture. A better method, though more expensive, is a spring-loaded puncture device (Figure 3.21). These devices hide the blade in a plastic holder so the patient cannot see the blade during the puncture. The plastic device lies on the skin, and the trigger is depressed. The spring forces the blade into the skin rapidly and then retracts. The rapid puncture and the invisible blade make the patient less apprehensive about skin punctures. The spring-loaded blades work by a guillotine action, a slicing motion. Devices can be purchased that puncture no more than 2.4 mm for newborn heelsticks. Other devices vary in depth for finger sticks of different-age patients. What should be avoided when collecting samples for laboratory specimens are the devices on the market for diabetic at-home blood glucose monitoring. These devices are excellent for their purpose but do not provide a blood flow of more than one or two drops of blood. This is not adequate blood flow for the sample size needed for most laboratory testing.

The devices used for collecting, processing, and transporting microcollections depend on the laboratory testing being performed. This discussion of devices here is not exhaustive. As the phlebotomist works in different laboratories, some specialized devices may also be used. Most of the microcollection equipment is intended for one-time use, to be disposed of later as hazardous waste.

Disposable calibrated micropipettes are thin-bore devices much like small glass soda straws that draw the blood up to a certain line on the glass. The line on the glass indicates the calibration for an amount drawn from 1 to 200 microliters. They are generally used for measurement of an amount of blood and then transferred to a container or solution. The blood draws up into the tube because of **capillary action.** Capillary action is the adhesive molecular force between liquid and solid materials that draws liquid into narrow-bore capillary tubes. The capillary action of a tube is enhanced if the tube is slanted in a semihorizontal direction as the blood is being drawn into the tube.

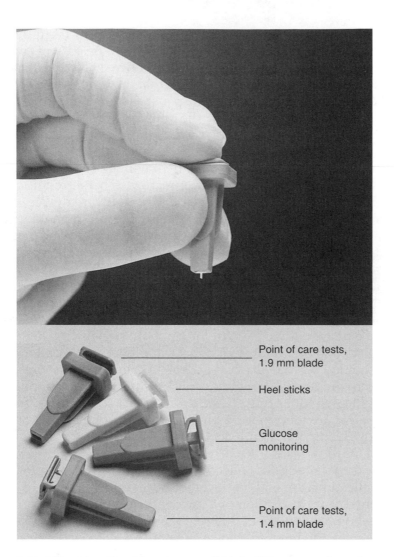

Point of care tests,
1.9 mm blade

Heel sticks

Glucose
monitoring

Point of care tests,
1.4 mm blade

Figure 3.21 *Microtainer Brand lancets are available in different types for various purposes. To use, hold lancet on skin, and depress plunger with index finger to make puncture. Immediately release plunger while holding lancet on site. Discard lancet after use in biohazard container. (Courtesy of Becton Dickinson Vacutainer Systems.)*

Glass has been the material for the micropipettes, but plastic or a plastic coating over the glass is now preferred. The glass has a tendency to break and cut the phlebotomist, exposing the phlebotomist to the patient's blood. The plastic micropipettes reduce the possibility of an accidental exposure.

Similar to calibrated micropipettes are microhematocrit capillary tubes. These tubes are narrow-bore pipettes primarily

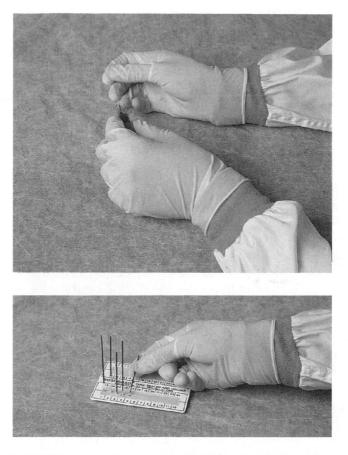

Figure 3.22 *(A) Filling a microhematocrit tube with blood by capillary action. (B) Sealing the microhematocrit tube with sealing clay. Note. From* Comprehensive Medical Assisting, Administrative and Clinical Competencies *(p. 850), by W. Lindh, M. S. Pooler, D. C. Tamparo, and J. U. Cerrato, 1998, Albany, NY: Delmar Publishers. Copyright 1998 by Delmar Publishers. Reprinted with permission.*

intended for determining packed red cell volume in microsamples. Once filled, the tubes are sealed and then are centrifuged in a special centrifuge that packs the formed elements of the blood. This packed red cell volume is then read on a scale that gives the packed volume as a percentage of the total. The result is the hematocrit of the patient. Since the volume is read on a special sliding scale, the total volume in the tube is not important. The volume required for the tube is between 50 and 75 microliters (Figure 3.22).

Blood gas collection pipettes collect skin puncture whole blood specimens under anaerobic conditions for blood gas determinations. The tubes vary in size but draw 50–250 microliters of volume. The amount of draw needed depends on the instrument used in the blood gas testing. The tubes contain heparin to keep the blood from clotting and generally a small magnetic stirrer, known as a **flea,** slides into the tube to maintain a mixed sample. The tubes are plugged with sealant putty or caps to maintain anaerobic conditions. Caraway or Natelson pipettes are general-purpose microcollection tubes that have a tapered end and are supplied with and without anticoagulant. They contain no markings to specify a volume and are used for the collection of skin puncture blood and the transfer to another container.

The process of collection and transfer of blood samples has been simplified with the use of noncapillary plastic microcollection devices. These devices consist of small round bottomed nonsterile plastic tubes. They include a means for filling, measuring, color coding for the proper anticoagulant, stoppering, centrifugation, and storage. The color coding matches the coding on the anticoagulant tubes: lavender is EDTA, green is heparin, and red gives a serum sample. The serum tubes can contain the thixotropic separator gel that separates the serum from the cells after centrifugation. Samples collected for bilirubin are collected in an amber tube that protects the blood from light. If a bilirubin specimen is not protected from light, the bilirubin level of the blood in the tube will rapidly decrease. The key to accurate test results after the collection of all microcollection specimens is a free-flowing sample. As the drop of blood forms, it is touched by the collection cap that consists of a scoop or tubing device in the cap. The blood then flows into the bottom of the tube. The tubes hold approximately 600 microliters of blood. The tubes go by a variety of brand names such as Microtainer or Microvette (Figure 3.23).

With some microcollections the phlebotomist is required to set up the test at the patient's bedside by collecting the sample and then making dilutions of the sample. A micropipette and dilution system are used to make this task easier (Figure 3.24). The brand name for this type of system is the Unopette system, manufactured by Becton Dickinson. The system consists of a plastic reservoir that contains a premeasured amount of **diluent** or **reagent,** a capillary pipette that fits into a plastic holder, and a pipette shield. The reservoir is punctured to open access to the reagent. Blood is drawn into the pipette. The filled pipette is rinsed to dilute the blood in the reagent. These devices are used for such tests as platelet counts, hemoglobin determinations, and white blood cell (WBC) and red blood cell (RBC) counts.

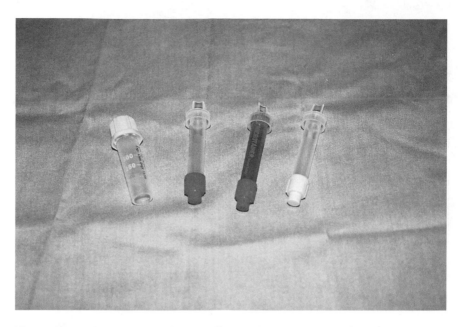

Figure 3.23 *Microtainer Brand microcollection devices. (Courtesy of Becton Dickinson Vacutainer Systems.)*

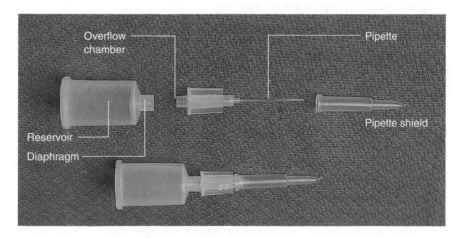

Figure 3.24 *Parts of a disposable Unopette blood-diluting unit: (A) unassembled Unopette unit and (B) assembled unit. Note. From* Comprehensive Medical Assisting, Administrative and Clinical Competencies *(p. 856), by W. Lindh, M. S. Pooler, D. C. Tamparo, and J. U. Cerrato, 1998, Albany, NY: Delmar Publishers. Copyright 1998 by Delmar Publishers. Reprinted with permission.*

```
PROCEDURE 3.1
```

COLLECTING A UNOPETTE BLOOD SAMPLE

Principle:

Properly and safely collect a blood sample into a Unopette blood-diluting device to determine either a platelet count, WBC count, or RBC count.

Materials:

Gloves
Hand disinfectant
Materials for capillary puncture
Unopette device
70 percent alcohol
Biohazard container for sharps

Procedure:

1. Wash hands, or use hand disinfectant if handwashing facilities are not available.

2. Puncture diaphragm. Using the protective shield on the capillary pipette, puncture the diaphragm of the reservoir as follows:

   a. Place the reservoir on a flat surface. Grasping the reservoir in one hand, take pipette assembly in the other hand and push tip of pipette shield firmly through diaphragm in neck of reservoir, then remove.

   b. Remove shield from pipette assembly with a twist.

   c. Gloves must be worn before fingerstick of patient and during the remaining procedure.

3. Add sample. After fingerstick of the patient, and wiping away the first drop of blood, the capillary must be filled with whole blood and transferred to the reservoir as follows:

   a. Holding the pipette almost horizontally, touch tip of pipette to the blood from the finger puncture. Pipette will fill by capillary action. Filling is complete and will stop automatically when blood reaches end of capillary bore in neck of pipette.

   b. Wipe excess blood from outside of capillary pipette, making certain no sample is removed from capillary bore.

   c. Squeeze reservoir slightly to force out some air. Do not expel any liquid. Maintain pressure on reservoir.

continues

PROCEDURE 3.1 *continued*

> d. Cover opening of overflow chamber with index finger, and seat pipette securely in reservoir neck.
> e. Release pressure on reservoir. Then remove finger from pipette opening. Negative pressure will draw blood into diluent.
> f. Squeeze reservoir gently two or three times to rinse capillary bore, forcing diluent into, but not out of, overflow chamber. Pressure is released each time to return the mixture to the reservoir.
> g. Place index finger over upper opening, and gently invert five to six times to thoroughly mix blood with diluent.
> h. Label the specimen and take to the laboratory.
> 4. Sources of error.
>> a. Squeezing the reservoir and spilling some of the liquid will give an inaccurate result.
>> b. While wiping the outside of the capillary pipette, any blood drawn out of the tube will lower the expected results.
>> c. Not wiping the blood from the outside of the capillary pipette will increase the expected results.
>> d. Bubbles in the capillary pipette or incomplete filling of the capillary pipette will lower the expected results.
>> e. Using a reservoir that has a punctured diaphragm will give inaccurate results.

Diabetic patients often do their own puncturing and collection. The patient collects a sample on a reagent strip pad, which is read by a hand-held glucose meter (Figure 3.25). The instrumentation for home use is continuing to expand. Several meters are also available to test a patient's coagulation.

The last microcollection device we discuss is blood collection on filter paper for neonatal screening programs (Figure 3.26). Neonatal screening identifies genetic defects. The newborn is punctured in the heel, and the blood is dropped onto a filter paper card. The blood is allowed to dry, and the blood-saturated filter paper is sent to the laboratory for testing. The genetic disorders the infant is tested for are phenylketonuria, galactosemia, hypothyroidism, homocystinuria, maple sugar urine disease, and sickle cell disease/hemoglobinopathies. With early identification of these diseases, treatment lessens the disorder and often completely prevents it.

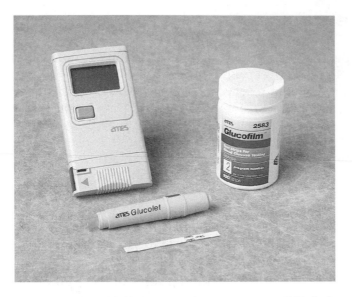

Figure 3.25 *A variety of hand-held glucose analyzers are now available for home or office use. These analyzers have become less expensive; however, the cost of the strips needed for the tests can be expensive, especially if used three times a day as recommended by most manufacturers. These analyzers do allow diabetics to safely test and track their blood glucose levels to help control diabetes. Note. From Comprehensive Medical Assisting, Administrative and Clinical Competencies (p. 961), by W. Lindh, M. S. Pooler, D. C. Tamparo, and J. U. Cerrato, 1998, Albany, NY: Delmar Publishers. Copyright 1998 by Delmar Publishers. Reprinted with permission.*

SPECIMEN COLLECTION TRAYS

The phlebotomist needs a specimen collection tray to hold all the equipment necessary for proper specimen collection. This tray will be taken to the patient's room so the phlebotomist is prepared for whatever procedure is performed. These trays vary depending on the type of collections usually done or the type of hospital or laboratory where the phlebotomist works. In some cases, a tray will not be adequate, and the phlebotomist will need to have a stocked cart to roll from room to room. The tray is usually preferred because it is more portable and can be taken upstairs to avoid a long wait at the elevator. The trays come in a variety of different sizes and shapes to better fit the phlebotomist's preference and needs (Figure 3.27).

The phlebotomist's tray should include at least the following:

1. Alcohol swabs.
2. Gauze squares or cotton balls.
3. Evacuated tube holders.

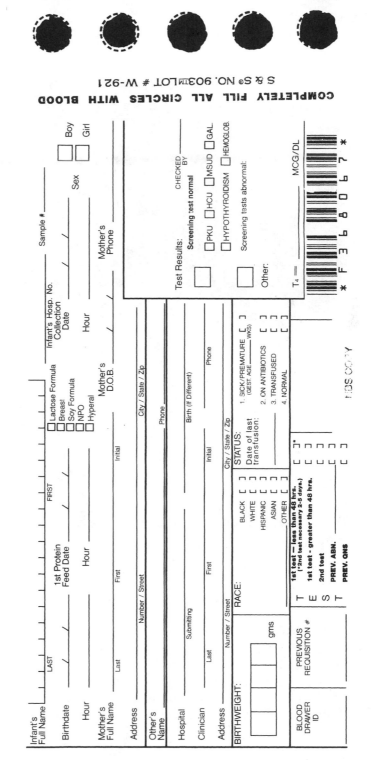

Figure 3.26 *Newborn screen card.*

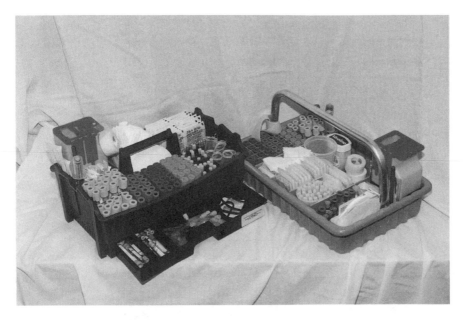

Figure 3.27   *Stocked phlebotomy trays. Note. From* Comprehensive Medical Assisting, Administrative and Clinical Competencies *(p. 829), by W. Lindh, M. S. Pooler, D. C. Tamparo, and J. U. Cerrato, 1998, Albany, NY: Delmar Publishers. Copyright 1998 by Delmar Publishers. Reprinted with permission.*

4. Assorted evacuated tubes.
5. Syringes.
6. Various-size syringe and evacuated tube needles.
7. Butterfly collection sets.
8. Lancets.
9. Microcollection equipment.
10. Tourniquets.
11. Disposable gloves.
12. Sharps container.
13. Marking pen.
14. Ammonia capsule.
15. Biohazard sharps container.

REVIEW QUESTIONS

Multiple Choice

Choose the one best answer.

1. 10 milliliters (ml) is the same as
   a. 1 liter
   b. 10 deciliters
   c. 10 cubic centimeters (cc)
   d. none of the above

2. Which needle has the smallest bore?
   a. 16-gauge needle
   b. 20-gauge needle
   c. 21-gauge needle
   d. 23-gauge needle

3. A short draw with a sodium citrate tube will lead to a
   a. prolonged APTT and prolonged PT
   b. shortened APTT and shortened PT
   c. prolonged APTT and shortened PT
   d. have no effect on the APTT or the PT

4. Which of the following anticoagulants prevent coagulation of the blood by removing calcium through the formation of insoluble calcium salts?
   a. EDTA
   b. oxalate
   c. sodium citrate
   d. heparin
   e. all the above
   f. a, b, and c

5. An anticoagulant is an additive placed in evacuated tubes in order to
   a. dilute the blood prior to testing

   b. ensure the sterility of the tube
   c. make the blood clot faster
   d. prevent the blood from clotting

6. A green-stoppered evacuated tube contains what kind of anti-coagulant?
   a. citrate
   b. fluoride
   c. heparin
   d. no additive

7. When serum is needed for testing, blood must be collected in which of the following colored tubes?
   a. blue
   b. green
   c. lavender
   d. red

8. Unsterile tubes may cause the following problem(s)
   a. false-positive blood cultures
   b. infect the patient through back flow
   c. short draws
   d. both a and b

9. The tourniquet should be applied how many inches above the proposed venipuncture site?
   a. 1–2 inches
   b. 3–4 inches
   c. 4–5 inches
   d. 5–6 inches

10. Leaving the tourniquet on a patient's arm for an extended length of time before drawing blood may cause
   a. hemoconcentration
   b. specimen hemolysis
   c. stress
   d. bruising

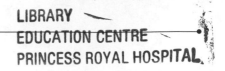

Critical Thinking

1. Explain the method that is used to prevent blood in the anticoagulant tubes from clotting.

2. How would a PT result be affected if the tube were only half full?

3. A physician calls and says that all the blood glucose results for his patients—from whom blood is drawn in his office and then sent to the laboratory—show low blood sugar. There must be a problem with the laboratory instrument. What would you investigate to resolve his problem?

4. You did a fingerstick on a patient and cannot seem to get enough blood. This patient is a construction worker with large, callused hands. What could be the problem?

BIBLIOGRAPHY

Lindh, W., Pooler, M. S., Tamparo, C. D., & Cerrato, J. U. (1998). *Comprehensive medical assisting, administrative and clinical competencies.* Albany, NY: Delmar.

National Committee for Clinical Laboratory Standards. (1992). *Blood collection on filter paper for neonatal screening programs* (2nd ed.). Approved Standard. NCCLS Document LA4-A2. Villanova, PA: Author.

National Committee for Clinical Laboratory Standards. (1990). *Devices for collection of skin puncture blood specimens* (2nd ed.). Approved Standard. NCCLS Document H14-A2. Villanova, PA: Author.

National Committee for Clinical Laboratory Standards. (1991). *Evacuated tubes for blood specimen collection.* Approved Standard. NCCLS Document H1-A3. Villanova, PA: Author.

National Committee for Clinical Laboratory Standards. (1991). *Procedures for the collection of diagnostic blood specimens by skin puncture* (3rd ed.). Approved Standard. NCCLS Document H4-A3. Villanova, PA: Author.

National Committee for Clinical Laboratory Standards. (1998). *Procedures for the collection of diagnostic blood specimens by venipuncture* (4th ed.). Approved Standard. NCCLS Document H3-A4. Villanova, PA: Author.

Wedding, M. E., & Toenjes, S. A. (1992). *Medical laboratory procedures.* Philadelphia: F. A. Davis.

Chapter 4

PHLEBOTOMY TECHNIQUE

O B J E C T I V E S

After studying this chapter, you should be able to:

1. Explain the three skills used in collecting blood.
2. Explain the importance of correct patient identification, complete specimen labeling, and proper accessioning.
3. List the components necessary for proper specimen labeling.
4. List four common venipuncture sites.
5. List four techniques that can make veins easier to feel.
6. Describe the step-by-step procedure for drawing blood.
7. List four ways to prevent hemolysis during venous collection.
8. Explain hemoconcentration and how to prevent it.
9. Explain the four precautions in blood collection.
10. Locate veins in the feet and ankles, and explain why they are not recommended for routine use.
11. Explain how to handle different patient reactions to venipuncture.
12. Discuss the three blood collection alternatives when a patient has an IV running in one arm.

13. Describe the proper technique for drawing from an indwelling line.

14. Describe the equipment used and preparation of equipment for arterial puncture.

15. Describe the Allen test.

16. Locate the four arterial sites and explain the order of preference for arterial puncture.

17. Explain the proper procedure for handling arterial blood.

K E Y   T E R M S

Aliquot	Part of the whole specimen that has been taken off for use or storage.
Arteriospasm	Reflex condition of the artery in response to pain or anxiety.
Cannula	Device used for access for dialyzing and for blood drawing in kidney patients.
Edema	Abnormal accumulation of fluid in the tissues resulting in swelling.
Fistula	Artificial shunt connection done by surgical procedure to fuse the vein and artery together. Used for dialysis only.
Hematoma	Leakage of blood out of the vein during or after venipuncture that causes a bruise.

STEPS IN THE BLOOD COLLECTION TECHNIQUE

Venipuncture is a detailed procedure requiring careful attention to each of the following steps:

1. Prepare accessioning order for the patient.
2. Greet and identify patient.
3. Verify diet/drug restrictions.
4. Wash hands, assemble supplies, and inspect equipment.
5. Reassure the patient.

6. Position the patient.
7. Verify paperwork and tubes.
8. Apply tourniquet.
9. Perform venipuncture.
10. Fill the tubes (if syringe and needle are used).
11. Remove tourniquet.
12. Dispose of sharps in proper container.
13. Label tubes.
14. Chill specimen or protect from light (only for certain tests).
15. Eliminate diet restrictions.
16. Time-stamp or computer verify paperwork.
17. Send correctly labeled tubes to proper laboratory departments.

Little attention is often given to these steps that are necessary for collecting a blood specimen. Our state-of-the-art sophisticated laboratory technology is often riddled with errors because of misidentification and poor sample collection techniques. All of the steps must be followed without deviation.

APPROACHING THE PATIENT

The phlebotomist uses three skills when contacting patients for phlebotomy: social (interpersonal), clerical, and technical.

Social skills are important. Always be polite and friendly with the patients even if they are rude or inconsiderate. Patients are often angry about their condition or fearful of the procedure and take it out on the first person they see. The phlebotomist could just be waking them up or could be entering the room right after the doctor gave them bad news. Whatever a patient says, it is inappropriate to counter with unprofessional remarks. The easiest way to defuse an upset patient is to be as polite as possible and explain that the doctor's orders need to be carried out. This social skill was outlined in the discussion of professionalism and a code of ethics in Chapter 1.

As the laboratory representative, the reputation of the entire laboratory rests with the phlebotomist. The patient's response to how well the laboratory performed while the patient was in the hospital is not influenced by the sophisticated instrumentation used to test the specimens. The response to friends and neighbors could be, "The blood drawers were the best I had ever seen. They were polite, skilled, and very gentle." The finest social skill guarantees this response from each patient.

Clerical skills are used constantly and contribute to the most errors in the health care setting. For the phlebotomist, the clerical skill is as simple as drawing the correct patient's blood and labeling it with the correct name. Sounds simple, but numerous errors occur in this one area. An error can have devastating effects. The wrong patient could be drawn for a transfusion of blood. The blood would be labeled with the name of the patient you were supposed to draw, but the blood in the tube would not be of that patient. The preparation of the blood for transfusion (crossmatch) would not be done on the correct blood. The patient could then receive units of blood that were not compatible. The side effects of such an error could be kidney failure or death.

Here is another example of a clerical error. The right patient was drawn for a blood glucose and the correct result was reported to the nursing unit. But the nurse misread the result and gave the wrong dosage of insulin. Clerical errors can occur at any step during the care of a patient. The phlebotomist does not want to be the cause of an error. The phlebotomist's errors are usually restricted to patient misidentification or mislabeling of a blood sample. Eight percent of errors in patient name, age, sex, and identification numbers are undetected despite many checking procedures. How to avoid these errors and develop an error-free clerical skill is discussed in the next section, "Patient Identification."

Technical skills mean obtaining blood successfully with minimal pain. They consist of whatever method is used to complete the procedure: venipuncture, arterial sample, or micro-collections through skin puncture.

Social, clerical, and technical skills are used in each patient contact and are intertwined in each step of taking a blood sample. The approach to the patient often determines the success of the venipuncture. The muscles of a tense patient tighten over the blood veins, making them more difficult to access. A relaxed patient is more cooperative and easier to draw.

PATIENT IDENTIFICATION

It cannot be repeated often enough that proper patient identification is essential to accurate patient testing. It does not matter how expensive or sophisticated the equipment the sample is tested on, the results will be wrong if the sample is not identified accurately.

Most patients have a hospital identification bracelet that includes their first and last names, hospital numbers (often two sets of numbers), birthdate, and physician. When the phlebotomist enters the room, do not say "Mr. Jones, I'm here to draw your blood" and assume if the patient says "yes" he is Mr. Jones. The patient will often have been asleep or not paying attention and will answer yes even if it is Mrs. Smith in the bed. Ask the conscious patient to state his or her full name. This lets patients realize someone is in the room and it gets them thinking so they will be awake when their blood is collected. The phlebotomist still needs to check the wristband to verify that the correct patient is being drawn even after the patient has stated his or her name. In addition to checking the patient's name, check the patient's identification numbers.

The identification numbers on the patient's wristband are compared to the name and numbers on the order form used in the health care institution. These order forms can be a manual requisition that is usually a multipart carbon form (Figure 4.1) or an adhesive computer label (Figure 4.2). The manual requisition is imprinted from an addressograph plate that prints the patient's name, identification numbers, physician, and room number. This plate is similar to a credit card plate, only it contains more information. The manual requisition can be handwritten. With either method, the test required is check marked or the required test is handwritten on the order form.

The computer label has several advantages. It lists the specific test that was ordered and the required specimen and specimen requirements. The barcode on the label contains information that can be used when running the test on the laboratory instruments. The barcode will tell the instrument what test to run, what patient the test is on, and other information that might be pertinent. The label is usually adhesive so it can be attached directly to the tube. Smaller labels can also be printed at the same time for smaller **aliquot** specimens. The computer has multiple other advantages in timing the print of orders, sorting lists of orders for one patient at one time, and speeding entry of draw times and test results. Most hospitals use some type of computer system for test ordering and result reporting. The computer labels print off in a roll where one label follows the other. Having two labels attached as in Figure 4.2 require special attention. One label must be carefully compared to the other to ensure that each label is for the same person, date, and time. Identifying patients by the computer labels and ensuring that each label used is for that patient requires using the following procedure:

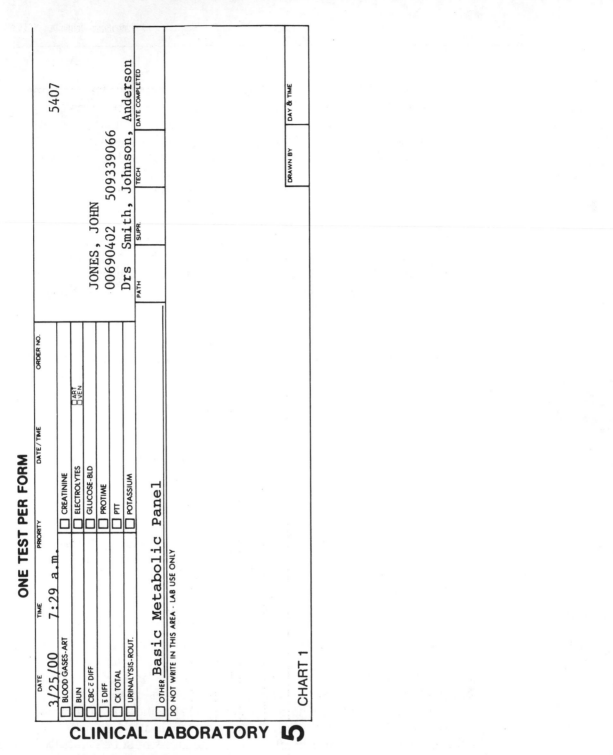

Figure 4.1 *Manual requisition.*

132

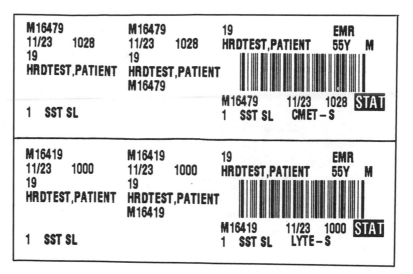

Figure 4.2 *Computer labels.*

PROCEDURE 4.1

PATIENT IDENTIFICATION

Principle:

To ensure that blood is collected from the correct person.

Procedure:

1. Approach the patient in a professional and courteous manner.
2. Collect all equipment and patient labels needed for only that venipuncture and take to patient's bedside.
3. Use the band identification procedure to ensure proper patient identification.
4. Perform a band identification procedure by doing either a label-to-label check or a band-to-label check.
   a. For a label-to-label check, compare the patient's first and last name and hospital registration number on the first label to the band to be sure they are exactly the same. Then compare the first label to each following label.
   b. For a band-to-label check, compare the patient's first and last name and hospital registration number on every label to the band.

continues

PROCEDURE 4.1 *continued*

5. After ensuring you have the correct patient, perform the venipuncture.

6. Perform band identification a second time using one of the methods in step 4.

7. Read each label as it is attached to the tube before leaving the bedside.

8. If computer labels are unavailable, labeling of the tubes may be done by (a) addressograph labels or (b) handwriting the patient's complete first and last name, hospital registration number(s), room number, date, and time of draw as required by the test.

9. Write the first and last initial of the phlebotomist on each specimen label.

10. If the patient does not have an identification band on his or her wrist or ankle, or if the identification band is not correct, notify the nurse or nursing unit secretary. *Do not draw blood unless the patient is wearing a correct identification band.*

11. All three identification checks are required: one verbal name and two identification band checks.

12. In some institutions you may be required to have the patient spell his or her last name.

13. If you suspect a labeling error, notify the supervisor.

ACCESSION NUMBER AND SPECIMEN IDENTIFICATION

Each request for a blood specimen may include an accession number: a number to identify all paperwork and supplies associated with each patient. This unique number can be used to trace back that specimen and patient. It ensures accurate and prompt processing of various forms required when performing a venipuncture and analyzing the results. A computerized system will generate the accession number when the specimen request is ordered in the computer. This number or letters and number are unique for that specimen and will be used in tracking the specimen, entering results of the test(s) on the specimen, and checking or reporting of the patient results. The blood request forms should include the following information:

1. Patient's name and age from ID plate or wristband.
2. Identification number.
3. Date and time the specimen is obtained.
4. Name or initials of person who obtains the specimen.
5. Accessioning number.
6. Physician's name.
7. Department for which work is being done.
8. Other useful information, for example, special comments: unusual sampling site, drawn near an IV site.

The blood is drawn and processed by institutional policy. Most health care areas do not label the tubes before the blood sample is drawn. Outpatient and inpatient specimens are labeled after the specimen is drawn and before the phlebotomist leaves the patient. In each case there is a potential for a clerical error. Each tube and label must be checked to ensure that proper identification is completed.

The American Association of Blood Banks (1996) sets the standards for labeling of blood bank specimens. As quoted in their technical manual:

> The intended recipient and the blood sample shall be positively identified at the time of collection. Blood samples shall be obtained in stoppered tubes identified with a firmly attached label bearing at least the recipient's first and last names, identification number, and the date. The completed label shall be attached to the tube before leaving the side of the recipient, and there must be a mechanism to identify the person who drew the blood.

The phlebotomist initials the label attached to the tube to identify himself or herself as the person who drew the blood. With computerized systems the phlebotomist also verifies in the computer who drew the sample.

POSITIONING THE PATIENT

The position of the patient is critical in proper blood collection. Proper comfortable positioning of the patient helps the patient feel more at ease, and the phlebotomist is better able to perform the venipuncture. The patient must be in a seated or reclined position before any attempt is made to draw blood. Do not allow patients to sit on a tall stool or stand while drawing blood. There is always the possibility patients will faint (syncope) and injure themselves. The sitting position requires a chair with adequate arm supports that are adjustable for the best venipuncture position. The reclined position is the ideal position from which to draw the patient. A pillow may be required to help support the patient's arm and keep it straight for easier venous access. Have patients lie down whenever they indicate they are apprehensive or have fainted in the past while having their blood drawn.

SELECTING THE APPROPRIATE VENIPUNCTURE SITE

The appropriate venipuncture site can vary depending on the patient. The site to check first is the upper region of the arm. The primary vein used in the upper arm is the median cubital vein, usually the prominent vein in the middle of the bend of the arm (Figure 4.3). The basilic, cephalic, or median veins can be used as a second alternative. These veins may not be accessible or may not be prominent enough to obtain a blood sample. The next step is to go to the back of the hand to obtain venous access. The veins in the back of the hand have the tendency to roll more than the arm veins because they are not supported by as much tissue and are near the surface. To avoid this, hold (anchor) the vein in place with your index finger and thumb while you use a smaller gauge needle or a butterfly. The hand veins are ideal for a butterfly with a 23-gauge needle. The butterfly can have a syringe attached to it or an evacuated tube holder attached. If the syringe is attached, careful slow pulling on the syringe will obtain the blood sample without collapsing the vein or hemolyzing the blood. For use of the evacuated tube holder, only small pediatric tubes should be used to avoid collapsing the vein. The wrist veins are also an alternative but generally are much more painful than the other sites. The foot and ankle veins may also be used. Some hospitals have restrictions on the use of the foot or ankle veins, and the patient's physician must give permission to use them. These veins are often restricted because the physician is concerned about clots forming in the legs. The veins also may be used for heart bypass surgery and the veins cannot be damaged with needle punctures. The veins in the foot or ankle also have the tendency to roll.

The order for checking for the best available site is (1) upper arm, (2) hand, (3) wrist, and (4) ankle or foot. The patient's condition dictates the site to use. Sites that should be avoided are edematous arms, arms in casts, arms with IVs, cannulas,

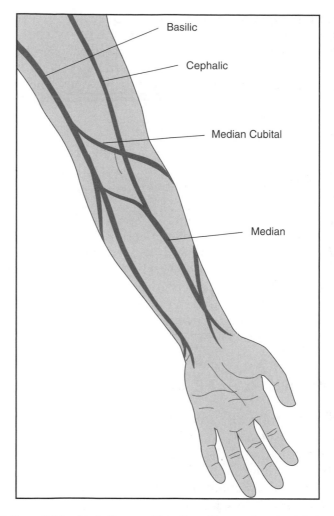

Basilic

Cephalic

Median Cubital

Median

Figure 4.3 *Superficial veins in the arm. Note. From* Comprehensive Medical Assisting, Administrative and Clinical Competencies *(p. 824), by W. Lindh, M S. Pooler, D. C. Tamparo, and J. U. Cerrato, 1998, Albany, NY: Delmar Publishers. Copyright 1998 by Delmar Publishers. Reprinted with permission.*

fistulas, extensive scarring such as burns, hematomas, or the arm on the side of a mastectomy. **Edematous** arms are swollen because of fluid in the tissue. The veins will not be prominent, and the tourniquet will be ineffective due to the swelling. Placement of the tourniquet has the potential for tissue damage and leaves a temporary indentation in the arm. Optimally, a patient on IV therapy should have specimens collected from the opposite arm. If this is impossible, other alternatives discussed later must be used. Blood should never be collected above the IV site. Cannulas and fistulas are devices that have been placed in the arm. Venipunctures should be performed from the opposite arm. Areas of scarring are also to be avoided because of possible injury to the patient or excessive pain. Specimens collected from a hematoma area may cause erroneous test results. If another vein site is not available, the specimen is collected distal from the hematoma. Because of the potential for harm to the patient due to lymphostasis, the arm on the side of a mastectomy should be avoided. If the patient has had a double mastectomy, a physician should be consulted prior to drawing the blood.

Often the site you draw from is determined by whatever site you feel is best to obtain the amount of blood you need. First look at both arms. If you find nothing that feels like a good vein, then check the back of the hand, followed by the wrist. The next alternative is to have a more experienced phlebotomist check or if possible draw the sample from a fingerstick. If all of these alternatives fail to obtain a blood specimen, consider obtaining permission to draw from the foot.

PERFORMING A SAFE VENIPUNCTURE

The first step in collecting a venous blood sample is to find the site that will give the best blood return. A tourniquet, as explained in Chapter 3, constricts the flow of blood and helps fill the veins with blood. The tourniquet should be placed 3–4 inches above the proposed site. The phlebotomist then looks for a vein. The term *look* is often misused in selecting a vein. Actually a vein is being felt for. The vein must be felt for with the tip of the index or middle fingers. Palpate and trace the path of the vein several times. Avoid using the thumb because it has a pulse and is not as sensitive as the rest of the fingers. The vein will feel soft and bouncy to the touch. Determine the roundness, direction, and depth of the vein. All veins do not go straight up and down the arm. They each follow different angles or cross the arm going side to side. If no veins become prominent, retie the tourniquet slightly tighter but not so tight as to stop the flow of arterial blood into the arm. An alternative is to use a blood pressure cuff instead of a tourniquet. The blood pressure cuff should be between 90 and 100 mm Hg. This will provide a wider band of constriction on the arm to make the veins prominent. The difficulty is releasing the blood pressure cuff rapidly enough at the completion of the venipuncture to prevent bruising.

If the "vein" you feel pulsates, it is an artery in the patient's arm and should not be punctured. Tendons may also be deceptive and appear as a vein. But they do not have the soft bouncy feel and are hard to the touch. Puncturing a tendon gives no blood return and is painful to the patient. There are also nerves that run the length of the arm. The nerves cannot be seen or felt, but by avoiding deep probing venipunctures, the chance of touching a nerve is diminished. If the patient complains about the venipuncture hurting excessively, it is best to stop and try another site.

A safe and accurate venipuncture often depends on the patient restrictions. Some tests require that the patient fast and/or eliminate certain foods before any blood samples can be taken. Time and diet restrictions vary according to the test. The patient may also be on certain drug restrictions. Collection is specifically timed so the patient has not received any medications (see "Timed Specimens" in Chapter 6).

Before a venipuncture can be performed, all supplies and equipment must be assembled. It is best to prepare everything before greeting the patient. Locate exactly what tubes you need and any special equipment that might be necessary. The patient must be confident in the phlebotomist's abilities. It creates insecurity if the phlebotomist has to leave the patient to check on what tube needs to be drawn or to go back and get something else. It is best to go over the list of tests to draw and even write down what tube is needed for what test. Ask questions before entering the room to avoid interruptions in obtaining the blood sample.

As the patient is drawn, be sure you can reach the tubes you need without crossing over the patient or stretching and possibly moving the needle after it is in the patient. The worst case is to not have everything within reach and the patient must be redrawn to finish all the blood work needed. Remember that occasionally a tube will not fill all the way. It is best to keep a few spare tubes or have the phlebotomy tray within reach.

Now it is time to greet the patient. The patient must be reassured that the procedure is going to be simple and only a slight inconvenience. Be friendly, outgoing, and talk to the patient, explaining the procedure. Do not tell the patient "This is not going to hurt." A needle is being placed in the patient's arm. The amount of pain varies with the patient. Warn the patient that he or she will feel a "little" stick. Usually the patient will not say a word during the puncture. The anticipation of having blood drawn is worse to many patients than the actual draw. Even if the patient does not respond, it is best to continue to explain as if the patient was alert. Comatose patients can often hear; they just are unable to communicate that they understand. Explaining what is being done often prevents the nonresponsive patient from moving when the blood is drawn. Conversation with all patients gives them the feeling someone cares about them. Friendly associates who are polite to patients are reassuring and caring. This concern for the patient brings more patients back to that health care institution than any other care anyone can offer.

Once the patient has been reassured and confidence gained, it is easy to get cooperation. While talking to the patient, verify the paperwork and tubes to be certain everything is correct. All types of clever comments can be made to check the patient's armband and labels. Ask to check the armband. When the armband matches, tell the patient he or she is the right person and wins the prize of a blood draw. The phlebotomist can be creative and come up with clever comments to gain the cooperation of the patient, making it easier to concentrate on the task of drawing blood.

SYRINGE VERSUS EVACUATED TUBE SPECIMEN COLLECTION

Now we come to the job of drawing blood from a patient. The patient has been identified, paperwork and tubes verified, equipment assembled, and the patient is comfortable. The next step is to tie the tourniquet (Figures 4.4–4.7). After tying the tourniquet, have the patient close his or her hand and then select a vein. Do not ask the patient to pump his or her fist. This can cause erroneous results. Place the patient's arm in a downward position if possible. After location of an acceptable vein, mentally map the location. Set mental crosshairs on it by visualizing the puncture site. For example, it might be referenced slightly over from this freckle and a little down from that wrinkle. The phlebotomist is often tempted to take a pen and mark an "x" at the intended puncture site, an unacceptable practice. Set those mental crosshairs for an accurate puncture. Now clean the site with a gauze pad soaked with 70 percent isopropyl alcohol solution. A commercially prepared alcohol pad or a pad with chlorhexidine, 0.5 percent, in alcohol may also be used. Cleanse the skin in a circular motion from the center to the outside. Allow the area to air dry to prevent hemolysis of the specimen

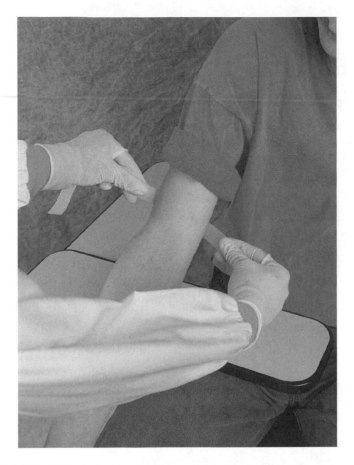

Figure 4.4 *Wrap the tourniquet around the arm 3 to 4 inches above the venipuncture site. Note. From* Comprehensive Medical Assisting, Administrative and Clinical Competencies *(p. 832), by W. Lindh, M. S. Pooler, D. C. Tamparo, and J. U. Cerrato, 1998, Albany, NY: Delmar Publishers. Copyright 1998 by Delmar Publishers. Reprinted with permission.*

and to prevent the patient from feeling a burning sensation during phlebotomy.

While the alcohol is drying, put on gloves if you haven't already done so. Some authorities suggest donning gloves first and then feeling for the vein. This is required procedure for the patient in isolation. For the nonisolation patient, gloves are not needed until there is a chance of coming in contact with blood and body fluid. The biggest deterrent to a phlebotomist wearing gloves is the inability to "feel" the vein. The time it takes for the alcohol to air dry on the arm is just enough time to put on gloves.

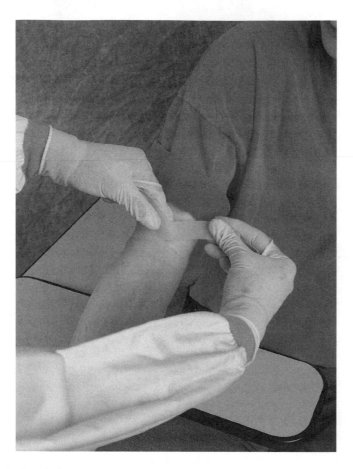

Figure 4.5 *Stretch the tourniquet tight, and cross the ends. Note. From* Comprehensive Medical Assisting, Administrative and Clinical Competencies *(p. 832), by W. Lindh, M. S. Pooler, D. C. Tamparo, and J. U. Cerrato, 1998, Albany, NY: Delmar Publishers. Copyright 1998 by Delmar Publishers. Reprinted with permission.*

To avoid forgetting where the collection site is, palpate the vein 1–2 inches above and below the intended puncture site. This helps you feel that the vein is located in a straight line. These points can be used to reset the mental crosshairs without contaminating the venipuncture site. Never palpate the vein directly on the puncture site without cleansing the skin again. If you have to cleanse the site again, then there will probably be a problem with prolonged tourniquet time and hemoconcentration. You must release the tourniquet and start again if the tourniquet has been on too long.

The syringe technique and the evacuated tube technique are the first two methods learned by the phlebotomist trainee. The

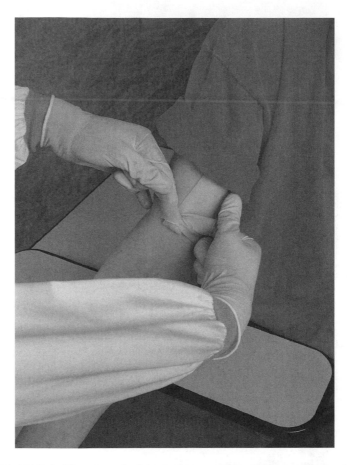

Figure 4.6 *While holding the ends tight, tuck one portion of the tourniquet under the other.* From Comprehensive Medical Assisting, Administrative and Clinical Competencies *(p. 832), by W. Lindh, M. S. Pooler, D. C. Tamparo, and J. U. Cerrato, 1998, Albany, NY: Delmar Publishers. Copyright 1998 by Delmar Publishers. Reprinted with permission.*

syringe technique is not as common as the evacuated system. But the techniques developed in the syringe method are building blocks for the evacuated tube technique and all other techniques.

Hold the syringe and needle system in your dominant hand, and cradle it on the four fingers. Place the thumb on top of the syringe. A right-handed person holds the syringe in the right hand, leaving the left hand to pull on the plunger. A left-handed person does the opposite. With the syringe held in this position, turn it slightly so the bevel of the needle is facing up. Puncturing a patient with the bevel down is painful to the patient. Grasp the patient's arm with the nondominant hand, using the thumb to

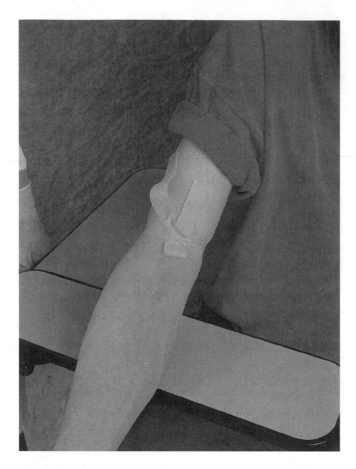

Figure 4.7 *Check that the tourniquet will not come loose. The ends of the tourniquet should be pointed upward. Feed for a vein. From* Comprehensive Medical Assisting, Administrative and Clinical Competencies *(p. 832), by W. Lindh, M. S. Pooler, D. C. Tamparo, and J. U. Cerrato, 1998, Albany, NY: Delmar Publishers. Copyright 1998 by Delmar Publishers. Reprinted with permission.*

draw the skin tight over the vein. The thumb should be 1–2 inches (2.0–5.0 cm) below the venipuncture site.

Line up the needle and syringe with the vein to be drawn. Rest the hand with the syringe gently on the patient's arm. Hold the hand in a position so that by tilting the point of the needle down slightly the needle will enter the skin at a 15-degree angle and about 0.5 cm below the point of the vein (Figure 4.8). Do not enter the vein at the exact point you felt the vein. The point you felt the vein is the point where the bevel of the needle must be under the skin. Push the needle into the skin. A sensation of resistance will

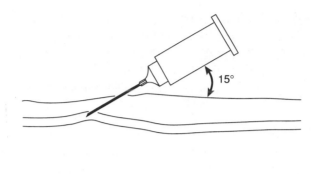

Figure 4.8 *Proper position of needle entering vein.*

be followed by easy penetration as the vein is entered. This is known as feeling the "pop." Once this point is reached, stop and do not move.

Take the nondominant hand and pull on the plunger of the syringe. Pull gently and only as fast as the syringe will fill with blood. Pulling too hard or fast will collapse the vein. If the vein does collapse, stop pulling on the plunger and let the vein refill with blood. If more blood is needed than the first syringe can hold, replace the syringe with another syringe. The needle should remain in the vein while this is being done. Place a clean gauze square under the needle to catch any blood while you make the change. Changing syringes creates a hazard and must be avoided if at all possible.

Ideally you should remove the tourniquet as soon as blood flow is established. This is not practical for the beginning phlebotomist. For a beginning phlebotomist, the act of removing the tourniquet may move the needle and/or vein just enough so no more blood can be obtained and the patient has to be redrawn. If the tourniquet is left on, the tourniquet must never be left on longer than one minute. The entire process should take less than one minute to complete. Always remove the tourniquet before removing the needle from the arm. Not removing the tourniquet before the needle is removed causes blood to be forced out of the needle hole and into the surrounding skin, resulting in a hematoma.

The syringe method of drawing venous blood is not the recommended method, since it is easier to use the evacuated system. The syringe is ideal for small blood samples in fragile surface veins or veins in the back of the hand. When a syringe is used, the blood obtained must be placed in appropriate containers. To place the blood in evacuated tubes, puncture the stopper with the syringe needle and allow blood to enter the tube until the flow stops. Do not remove the rubber stoppers. Running blood down the side of the tube after removing the stopper is not recommended because aerosols and splattering of blood can occur. Mix if any anticoagulant is present. Do not hold the tube in your hand as you puncture the stopper. There is the potential for missing the stopper or slipping off the stopper and puncturing yourself. The best method is to have the tubes in a test tube rack and then puncture the tubes using only one hand. The tube will fill itself. Do not force the blood into the tube. This technique maintains the proper ratio of blood to anticoagulant. The order of filling the tubes is important. The recommended order of fill from a syringe venipuncture is as follows:

1. Blood culture bottles or yellow-stoppered blood culture tube (sterile procedures).
2. Plain tube, nonadditive (e.g., red stopper).
3. Coagulation tube (e.g., light blue stopper).
4. Additive tubes:
    a. Gel separator tube.
    b. Heparin (e.g., green stopper).
    c. EDTA (e.g., lavender stopper).
    d. Oxalate/fluoride (e.g., gray stopper).

Fill the sterile collection bottles/tubes first to prevent bacterial contamination. To further prevent bacterial contamination, clean the tops of the bottles/tubes with alcohol before the rubber stopper is punctured. When the syringe system is used and a large specimen is taken, fill the coagulation tube(s) from the second syringe.

A detailed procedure for venipuncture with syringe is as follows:

PROCEDURE 4.2

VENIPUNCTURE BY SYRINGE

Principle:

To obtain venous blood acceptable for laboratory testing as required by a physician.

continues

PROCEDURE 4.2   *continued*

Specimen:

Venous blood collected to be aliquoted into evacuated tubes and/or special collection containers.

Materials:

Syringe, vary in size
Disposable needle for syringe, 21- or 22-gauge needle
Evacuated tube(s) or special collection tube(s)
Tourniquet
70 percent isopropyl alcohol swab
Gauze or cotton balls
Adhesive bandage or tape
Sharps container
Disposable gloves
Biohazard sharps container
Safety glasses and mask

Procedure:

1. Identify patient. *Inpatient:* Verify wrist band name and hospital number with computer label or requisition information. *Outpatient:* Ask patient his or her name, and verify with computer label or requisition information.
2. If a fasting specimen is required, ask the patient when he or she last ate. Explain procedure to the patient.
3. Wash hands. Open the sterile needle and syringe packages, attaching the needle if necessary.
4. Prevent the plunger from sticking by pulling it halfway out and pushing it all the way in one time.
5. Select the proper tube(s) to transfer the blood to after collection. Place in the proper order for filling.
6. Apply tourniquet.
7. Ask patient to close hand. The patient must not be allowed to pump the hand. Place the patient's arm in a downward position if possible.
8. Select a vein, noting the location and direction of the vein.
9. Clean venipuncture with 70 percent isopropyl alcohol swab.
10. Put on gloves while alcohol is drying. Do not touch venipuncture site.

continues

PROCEDURE 4.2 *continued*

11. Draw the patient's skin taut with your thumb. The thumb should be 1–2 inches below the puncture site.

12. With the bevel up, line up the needle with the vein and perform venipuncture. While securely grasping the syringe with one hand, use the other hand to slowly pull the plunger back until the desired amount of blood has been obtained.

13. Replace the syringe with another syringe if additional blood is needed. The needle should remain in the vein. Place a clean gauze under the needle during this procedure to catch blood while making the change.

14. Ask patient to open the hand.

15. Release tourniquet.

16. Lightly place gauze square or cotton ball above venipuncture site.

17. Remove needle from arm.

18. Apply pressure to the site for three to five minutes. The patient may assist if able.

19. Aliquot blood into appropriate tube(s). Puncture stopper of evacuated tube with syringe needle, and allow blood to enter tube until flow stops. Mix if any anticoagulant is present. If tube(s) are not evacuated-type tubes, remove needle by the needle unwinder on the sharps container or scoop needle cap up one-handed and then unscrew resheathed needle. Blood is then expelled into tube(s) until proper fill.

20. Dispose of needle and syringe in sharps container.

21. Recheck armband with labels or requisitions.

22. Label all tubes.

23. Apply adhesive bandage.

The evacuated tube system is an improvement over the syringe method but maintains many similarities. With the syringe method, as the syringe plunger is pulled, a vacuum is created. The evacuated method has the vacuum already in the tube. Another advantage of the evacuated tube system is that with multiple blood samples syringes do not need to be changed, just tubes.

The similarity of the evacuated tube system is that the holder and needle are held in the same manner as a syringe. A syringe is held in a manner to leave access to pull on the plunger. Access must be left in the evacuated system for one tube to be pulled out and another inserted. The hand that pulled on the plunger of the syringe is the hand that changes tubes with the evacuated system.

The procedure for venipuncture with the evacuated tube system follows the same steps as the syringe method with only slight variation:

PROCEDURE 4.3

VENIPUNCTURE BY EVACUATED TUBE METHOD

Principle:

To obtain venous blood acceptable for laboratory testing as required by a physician.

Specimen:

Venous blood collected by evacuated tubes. Volume of blood dependent on size of tube and test requirements.

Materials:

Evacuated tube holder
Disposable needle for evacuated system, 20-, 21- or 22-gauge needle
Evacuated tube(s) or special collection tube(s)
Tourniquet
70 percent isopropyl alcohol swab
Gauze or cotton balls
Adhesive bandage or tape
Sharps container
Disposable gloves
Biohazard sharps container
Safety glasses and mask

Procedure:

1. Identify patient. *Inpatient:* Verify wristband name and hospital number with computer label or requisition information. *Outpatient:* Ask patient his or her name and verify with computer label or requisition information.
2. If a fasting specimen is required, ask the patient when he or she last ate. Explain the procedure to the patient.

continues

PROCEDURE 4.3   *continued*

3. Collect equipment. Wash hands.

4. Break needle seal. Thread the appropriate needle into the holder using the needle sheath as a wrench.

5. Before using, tap all tubes that contain additives to ensure that all the additive is dislodged from the stopper and wall of the tube.

6. Insert the tube into the holder until the needle slightly enters the stopper. Avoid pushing the needle beyond the recessed guideline, because a loss of vacuum may result. If the tube retracts slightly, leave it in the retracted position.

7. Apply tourniquet.

8. Ask patient to close hand. The patient must not be allowed to pump the hand. Place the patient's arm in a downward position to prevent reflux or "backflow" of the blood from the tube into the venous system.

9. Select a vein, noting the location and direction of the vein.

10. Clean venipuncture with 70 percent isopropyl alcohol swab.

11. Put on gloves while alcohol is drying. Do not touch venipuncture site.

12. Draw the patient's skin taut with your thumb. The thumb should be 1–2 inches below the puncture site.

13. With the bevel up, line up the needle with the vein and perform venipuncture. Remove your hand from drawing the skin taut. Grasp the flange of the evacuated tube holder, and push the tube forward until the butt end of the needle punctures the stopper. You should not change hands while performing the venipuncture. The hand you perform the venipuncture with is the hand that holds the evacuated tube holder. The opposite hand manipulates the tubes.

14. Fill the tube until the vacuum is exhausted and blood flow into the tube ceases, ensuring the proper blood-to-anticoagulant ratio.

15. When the blood flow ceases, remove the tube from the holder. While securely grasping the evacuated tube holder with one hand, use the other hand to change the tubes. The sleeve re-covers the point, stopping the flow of blood until the next tube of blood is inserted.

16. Mix immediately after drawing each tube that contains an additive. Gently inverting the tube five to ten times provides adequate mixing without causing hemolysis.

17. To obtain additional specimens, insert the next tube into the holder and repeat the procedure with step 14.

18. Ask patient to open hand.

continues

PROCEDURE 4.3 *continued*

19. Release tourniquet.
20. Lightly place gauze square or cotton ball above venipuncture site.
21. Remove needle from arm. Be certain last tube drawn has been removed from the holder before removing needle. This will prevent dripping blood out of the tip of the needle.
22. Apply pressure to the site for 3–5 minutes. The patient may assist if able.
23. Dispose of needle in sharps container.
24. Recheck armband with labels or requisitions.
25. Label all tubes.
26. Apply adhesive bandage.

With multiple draws, the order of drawing the tubes is important. The recommended order of draw from a single venipuncture using the evacuated system is the same as with a syringe:

1. Blood culture bottles or yellow-stoppered blood culture tube (sterile procedures).
2. Plain tube, nonadditive (e.g., red stopper).
3. Coagulation tube (e.g., light-blue stopper).
4. Additive tubes:
   a. Gel separator tube.
   b. Heparin (e.g., green stopper).
   c. EDTA (e.g., lavender stopper).
   d. Oxalate/fluoride (e.g., gray stopper).

Fill the sterile collection bottles/tubes first to prevent bacterial contamination. To further prevent bacterial contamination, clean the tops of the bottles/tubes with alcohol before the rubber stopper is punctured.

The nonadditive tubes are drawn before the additive tubes to avoid contamination of the nonadditive tube. Cross contamination between additive tubes can occur, affecting the test results. The effect of the cross contamination is lessened by maintaining the order of draw. The coagulation tube (light-blue stopper) is often the second or third tube drawn. If the physician's order is for routine coagulation testing—prothrombin time (PT) and activated partial thromboplastin time (APTT)—then the first tube collected can be the light-blue-stoppered tube. For special coagulation testing (factor assays), a plain red tube of at least 7.0 ml volume must be drawn as a discard tube first. This discard tube eliminates possible thromboplastin contamination from the venipuncture site. Thromboplastin is a substance produced by the patient and released into the blood stream as a reaction to the venipuncture. In most testing, it has no effect. With special coagulation testing, there is an effect. The discard tube clears the thromboplastin from the bloodstream.

To remember the order of draw, remember the beginning and end of the order. Remember that the order begins with all sterile collections, then clot tubes, and ends with a gray tube. Tubes drawn between these draws are drawn in alphabetical order (blue-gel-green-lavender).

PATIENT REACTIONS

Patients can have a variety of reactions to having their blood drawn. The phlebotomist must anticipate these reactions and respond quickly and appropriately. The most common patient reaction is pain. The patient may indicate the venipuncture is painful. Try repositioning the needle slightly and releasing the tourniquet. Releasing the tourniquet often helps because the tourniquet may be pinching the arm and hurting instead of the needle. Avoid deep, probing venipunctures, since they go deeper into the skin and get closer to the nerves. If the pain persists, discontinue the venipuncture.

Syncope (fainting) is preceded by the patient turning pale, perspiring, and starting to breathe shallowly. This is followed by drooping eyelids, weak, rapid pulse, and finally unconsciousness. If a patient does faint, immediately remove the needle and stop the patient from getting hurt. The patient in a chair will have to be held there to keep from sliding out onto the floor. Lower the head and arms. Wipe the patient's forehead and back of the neck with a cold compress if necessary. Pass an ammonia inhalant under the patient's nose (the patient should respond by coughing). If the patient still does not respond, a physician must be notified. It is best to ask the patient prior to drawing the blood if he or she has had any reactions to having blood drawn. If the patient states he or she has fainted in the past, have the patient lie down before drawing the blood, which usually prevents the problem. Never draw a patient standing or sitting on a stool.

Having their blood drawn is so upsetting to some patients that they become nauseated and vomit. The patient may indicate that he or she feels sick. Make the patient as comfortable as possible, and instruct the patient to breathe deeply and slowly. Apply cold compresses to the patient's forehead. Give the patient an emesis basin, wastebasket, or container, and have facial tissues ready if the nausea does not diminish. Give the patient water to rinse out his or her mouth if vomiting does occur.

Patients can go into insulin shock/hypoglycemia because they have fasted. Diabetic patients need to regulate their diet and eat at specific times of the day. If a test is needed to be drawn while fasting, the patient breaks from his or her normal routine and does not eat breakfast before coming in to have blood drawn. The patient is one to two hours late eating breakfast and can go into insulin shock from low blood sugar. The first signs are a cold sweat and pale face similar to the signs of syncope. The patient becomes weak and shaky followed by sudden mental confusion that appears as an instant personality change. At this point the patient may indicate what is happening or lapse into unconsciousness. If the patient is conscious enough to swallow, a glass of orange juice or cola will help temporarily. Call a physician if the patient remains unconscious.

A patient who goes into convulsions becomes unconscious and exhibits violent or mild convulsive motions. Do not try to restrain the patient but move objects or furniture out of the way to prevent injury. Call the physician or nurse to help with the situation. The patient will usually recover within a few minutes and will be able to leave after a few minutes of rest.

Many individuals who come in to have their blood drawn have a health problem. A person with heart problems could go into cardiac arrest. The patient falls into unconsciousness, has no pulse or respiration, dialated eyes, and a blue or gray skin tone. Immediate cardiopulmonary resuscitation (CPR) is necessary to avoid patient death. Only persons certified to do CPR can perform this procedure. Most health care institutions call this occurrence a code or code blue. Each institution has a certain protocol to announce the code and call the code team that will take over in caring for the patient.

Upon completion of a venipuncture, a gauze square or cotton ball is placed on the puncture site to help stop the bleeding. Normally the bleeding will stop in approximately two minutes, the time it takes to label and initial the tubes that were drawn. Some patients have continuous bleeding at the venipuncture site for longer than five minutes. Continue to apply pressure to the site by wrapping a gauze bandage around the arm over a pad. Tell the patient to leave the bandage on for at least fifteen minutes, but as long as necessary to stop the bleeding.

A patient can react by leaking blood under the skin at the site of the venipuncture during or after the venipuncture. A **hematoma** (bruise) will result. The phlebotomist should use the major superficial veins for venipuncture. Only the uppermost wall of the vein should be punctured to prevent a hematoma. The puncture should not be so deep that the top and bottom wall of the vein are punctured. The puncture should be deep enough to fully penetrate the uppermost wall of the vein (partial penetration allows blood to leak around the puncture site). After any venipuncture, a small amount of pressure should be applied to the area. Place adequate cotton or gauze under the bandage to prevent bleeding.

Petechiae, small red dots that are indications of small amounts of bleeding under the skin surface, may be present on the skin surface of some patients. These are often the result of low platelet counts or other coagulation problems. The patient may bleed excessively after the venipuncture.

Some patients are allergic to tape or iodine. The patient will stop you as you try to put tape on the arm if he or she is allergic. Before you leave this patient, check that all bleeding has stopped and tell the patient to hold a cotton ball or gauze square on the puncture site. The gauze on cotton can be held in place with hypoallergenic tape. Blood cultures require iodine for cleansing the collection site. Before the phlebotomist uses iodine on a patient, the patient should be asked if he or she has any allergies.

Three characteristics of patient's blood can result in altered test results. The most frequently seen characteristic is hemolysis of the red blood cells. Hemolysis is a breaking or rupturing of the membrane of the red blood cells. The contents of the red blood cells then contaminate the serum or the plasma being tested. The serum or plasma appears red. The darker the red, the more cells that have been hemolyzed. The causes of hemolysis are: (1) drawing from a hematoma; (2) rupturing of the red blood cells by using a needle that is too small; (3) alcohol on the site of the venipuncture that enters the blood sample; (4) leakage of air and frothing of the blood through a needle not attached to the syringe tightly enough; (5) pulling back the plunger of the syringe too forcibly; and (6) temperature extremes. Blood left in a car could get too hot in the summer or freeze in the winter. In either case, the red blood cells will rupture.

A patient's serum or plasma that contains a large amount of bilirubin because of jaundice will have a yellow to orange color. The patient's skin may also have the same yellow to orange color. Serum or plasma with this coloration is called icteric. It is not caused by the phlebotomist's error, but results from the patient's condition.

A large amount of fats and lipids in a patient's blood gives the serum and plasma a white, milky color. This type of serum or plasma is known as lipemic. It, too, is the result of the patient's condition and not a phlebotomist's error. The lipemic appearance also may be due to the patient not having fasted.

THE FAILED VENIPUNCTURE

When you cannot obtain a blood sample, it may be necessary to change the position of the needle. Rotate the needle half a turn. The bevel of the needle may be against the wall of the vein. If the needle has not penetrated the vein far enough, advance it further into the vein. Only advance slightly. A small change makes the difference between a failed and a successful venipuncture. If the needle has penetrated too far into the vein, pull back a little. Always pull out slowly when the venipuncture has been unsuccessful. The blood will often start coming just as it seems the needle is ready to come out of the skin.

There are several reasons for venipuncture failure. The tube may have pulled back out of the holder. The tubes often will not stay pushed all the way into the holder while the blood is being collected. The tube slides back out, and then the tube stops filling with blood. A slight pressure holding the tube into the holder will remedy this problem. The tube being used may not have sufficient vacuum. Try another tube before withdrawing. The tourniquet could have been on too tight, stopping the flow of blood. Reapply the tourniquet loosely. An alternative to a tourniquet is a blood pressure cuff inflated to 90–100mm Hg. The cuff provides a larger surface area to apply pressure, and the pressure can be regulated. This often brings veins to the surface when other methods have failed.

Blood flow can also be stimulated by massaging the arm in an upward motion below the venipuncture site. Patting the venipuncture site can stimulate veins to be more prominent. If these techniques do not work, position the arm lower than the patient. Hang the patient's arm over the side of the bed, for example, causing the blood to pool more in the arm and make the veins more prominent.

Probing of the site is not recommended, because it is painful to the patient and may cause a hematoma. Use a vein in the opposite arm, or puncture a site below the first site. Never attempt a venipuncture more than twice. If a blood sample cannot be obtained in two tries, do a microcollection if possible, or have another person attempt the draw. Notify the patient's physician if two phlebotomists have been unsuccessful and a microcollection is not possible.

INTRAVENOUS AND INDWELLING LINES

Intravenous (IV) lines supply needed fluids and medicines to the patient. When an IV solution is being administered into one arm, blood should not be drawn from that arm. Blood drawn from the arm containing the intravenous solution has the potential to contaminate the blood specimen. These fluids and medicines can cause erroneous results in a blood sample. Intravenous lines are inserted into a vein. The site can be anywhere from the back of the hand to further up the arm. The IV sites are generally not placed in the upper area of the arm but any site below the upper arm. That makes the upper arm area very tempting to draw blood from because you can feel veins in the upper arm and the IV is in the lower part of the arm. Venous blood flow is flowing up the arm from the hand to the shoulder. The IV solution is flowing in that direction. Any blood drawn in a site above the IV will contain the IV solution. The IV solution will be in a high concentration because it has not had a chance to circulate through the body and distribute through the circulatory system. Therefore, the laboratory test results will be higher or lower depending on the contents of the IV solution.

If glucose is being tested in a patient who has a saline solution running in the IV, the value for the blood glucose will be less than actual due to the dilution. If a glucose solution is running in the IV, the value for the blood glucose will be increased due to the concentration of glucose solution. Test results are therefore erroneous and misleading to the physician. These erroneous results will cause the physician to treat the patient incorrectly.

To avoid this kind of error, look for a blood-drawing site in the opposite arm. Occasionally, an IV will be running in both arms and no site can be found except in the area of the IV. Satisfactory samples can be drawn below the IV by following several precautions. Ask the nurse to shut off the IV for at least two minutes before venipuncture. Apply the tourniquet below the IV site.

Select a vein other than the one with the IV. Perform the venipuncture. Draw 5 ml of blood, and discard this blood to clear any IV solutions from the arm before test samples are collected.

If the IV cannot be shut off, there are three options. First choice is to do a fingerstick if the tests ordered can be done by microcollection. Second, obtain permission from the physician to draw from the ankle or foot. The third option is to wait until the IV is taken out and then draw the blood sample.

To eliminate some of these problems, a new cooperation between the laboratory and nursing departments has started in many health care areas. Nurses are starting to draw more of the blood samples. To save the patient the discomfort of being punctured to start the IV and then punctured again to obtain the blood sample, the nurse inserts the IV needle and, before starting it, pulls a blood sample. This saves the patient a needle puncture and speeds the blood samples to the laboratory without the delay of waiting for the phlebotomist. No longer is the phlebotomist the only health care associate drawing blood from patients.

A variety of types of cardiovascular (arterial, central, venous) or umbilical lines are being used on patients. A line is a piece of tubing inserted into the patient's vein or artery. Through this line medications can be administered or blood samples can be taken. Obtaining blood specimens from indwelling lines or catheters can be a source of laboratory test errors if not collected properly.

To keep blood from clotting in the line, heparin or saline is used to flush the line. After blood is pulled from the line, heparin or saline is injected into the line until all the blood is pushed back into the patient. This keeps the line clear until the next blood sample needs to be taken. Any samples first taken from the line contain a mixture of blood and heparin or saline. At least 7 ml of blood must be discarded to clear all the heparin/saline. After the discard, the blood can be drawn as if you were drawing from a vein. Not discarding 7 ml of blood could cause erroneous results.

The method of drawing can be with a syringe or with an evacuated system. To draw from a line with the evacuated system, a *Luer adapter* (Figure 4.9) is used. A Luer adapter looks like an evacuated needle without the needle. The part that screws into the holder has the same needle and rubber sleeve. The needle that would normally be used on the patient is replaced with a port to fit in the line. The port can be fit into the line, and multiple tubes can be drawn. Once drawing is completed, the heparin/saline must be replaced in the line. In some states, the injection of heparin into the line by a phlebotomist is not permitted.

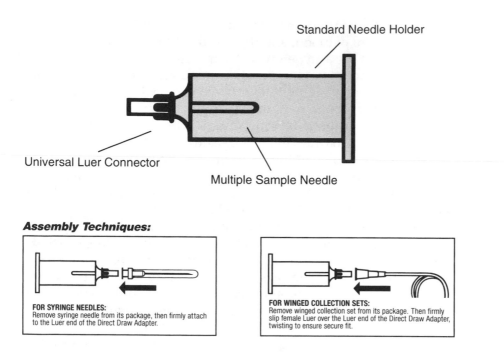

Figure 4.9 *Luer Adapter (direct draw adapter). (Courtesy of Becton Dickinson Vacutainer Systems.)*

Phlebotomists in some situations are drawing blood from lines, but usually nurses do this type of collection. The same limitations hold for accessing a **cannula**, a type of tubing connector used on kidney transplant or dialysis patients.

Some dialysis patients have fistulas. A **fistula** is an artificial shunt connection done by a surgical procedure to fuse together a vein and an artery. When encountering a patient with a fistula, specimens should be drawn from the opposite arm.

IDENTIFICATION OF THE SPECIMEN

Identification of the specimen is as important as the identification of the patient. If the correct patient was drawn but the specimen was misidentified, the patient could receive erroneous results. All specimens should be labeled before you leave the patient. Use the band identification procedure to ensure proper patient identification. The specimen is identified by using a computer label, addressograph label, or handwritten information on the tube. If there is more than one specimen to be labeled on a patient, check the labels so they all contain the same patient information. Do a label-to-label check. Compare the patient's first and last name and hospital registration number on the first label to the band to be sure they are exactly the same. Then compare the first label to each following label.

If computer or addressograph labels are unavailable, label the tubes by hand writing on each tube the following information:

1. Patient's complete first and last name.
2. Hospital registration number(s).
3. Room number.
4. Date and time of draw.
5. Phlebotomist's initials.

Recent advances in specimen identification include the use of computer bar codes to identify specimens and patients. The instruments doing the testing can read the bar codes. The results of the tests automatically enter into the patient's record without anyone entering results by hand onto a chart or into a computer. This is a computer interface of the instrument and the record-keeping computer. In actuality it is more complex than illustrated here. The purposes of the interface and use of bar codes is to speed computer entry of results and eliminate clerical errors.

CRITERIA FOR RECOLLECTION OR REJECTION OF A SPECIMEN

The one goal of the phlebotomist is to provide an acceptable specimen for laboratory testing as required by the physician. Certain general criteria must be followed for a specimen to be acceptable. If the criteria are not followed, the specimen must be rejected and recollected.

1. Each specimen must have its own label attached to the specimen's primary container.
2. Each specimen must have the test to be performed on the label (complete blood counts, cholesterol, etc.).
3. Labels must have the patient's complete name and hospital number.
4. Specimens in syringes with needles still attached are unacceptable.

5. Urine specimens must have the label on the container and not on the lid.

6. All specimens must be in their appropriate anticoagulant.

7. Anticoagulated blood collection tubes must be at least 75 percent full. All coagulation blood collection tubes must be at least 90 percent full.

8. Anticoagulated blood specimens must be free of clots.

9. Certain tests require specimens to be free of hemolysis and lipemia.

10. Blood specimens drawn above an IV site are unacceptable.

11. Urine specimens unrefrigerated for more than two hours or refrigerated for more than eight hours are unacceptable.

12. The specimen must be re-collected if the results are not consistent with previous results on the patient.

This list is not all-inclusive. The type of specimen acceptable and the volume required are determined by the procedure ordered. Re-collection is most often done to recheck results on a patient. When the results from one specimen change significantly from a previous specimen, the test is rechecked by either retesting the specimen or re-collecting the sample. This reconfirms the correct patient was drawn and/or the patient's test results did change significantly.

PRIORITIZING SPECIMEN COLLECTION

The phlebotomist is faced with the decision of which patient to draw first and which patients to draw later. Some hospitals allow tests to be ordered with different priorities. The stat test indicates the sample collection is critical to the immediate treatment of the patient. These specimens must be collected before other specimens. The as soon as possible (ASAP) order priority is sometimes used to indicate the specimen needs to be collected generally within an hour of the order time. Lesser priorities would be this A.M./P.M. or today.

Specimens that have a specific time to be drawn dictate the proper collection time and sequence. Stat specimens should always be collected first. After a stat specimen is collected, it must not be carried on the phlebotomist's tray while other less priority specimens are collected. The stat should be taken immediately to the appropriate laboratory.

Certain types of tests determine when the phlebotomist collects the specimen. In the blood test for ammonia, the specimen must be placed on ice and then delivered to the laboratory within twenty minutes of collection. If a phlebotomist has several patients to draw and one of those patients has an ammonia, the patient with the ammonia must be drawn last and then delivered to the laboratory. Each laboratory determines the priority for specimen collection.

ARTERIAL PUNCTURES

Arterial punctures are not for the beginning phlebotomist. Extensive observation and training in the technique should be completed before an arterial puncture is attempted. The patient could be seriously injured if the arterial sample is not collected correctly. Arterial punctures are used to obtain a specimen for blood gas analysis. The blood gas determines the effectiveness of a patient's ability to utilize oxygen and carbon dioxide. All living cells in the body must absorb oxygen and expel carbon dioxide. The dissolved oxygen in the blood is the PO_2. The dissolved carbon dioxide is the PCO_2. The pH of the blood is a measure of the acid–base balance of the blood. A pH of 7.40 is a perfect balance. The blood transports these dissolved gases to and from the cells. The arterial blood that has just left the heart and lungs has the highest concentration of oxygen. The arterial blood has a uniform composition of gases in all parts of the body. The venous blood gas varies depending on cell location. The muscular and metabolic activity of the cells varies the amount of gas the blood contains at different locations in the body. Due to the uniformity of the arterial blood gas, the arterial blood is the sample of choice for blood gas analysis.

Anxiety or excitement of the patient can alter the breathing pattern of the patient and change the composition of the blood gas. The blood gases are best during a period of *steady state*, when the patient is resting comfortably and has had no recent physical activity or treatments. A patient who fears needles and pain associated with arterial blood collection will change rapidly from this steady state. Some health care institutions use an anesthetic solution such as 0.5 percent lidocaine to numb the skin overlying the site before puncture. If this is done, a 1-ml syringe with 25-gauge needle is necessary for the injection. Numbing of the skin lessens the pain and prevents hyperventilation, breath holding, and anxiety. A stabilized breathing pattern gives more reliable results.

Improper transport and handling of blood gas samples can also alter the results rapidly. The specimen must be sealed and placed on ice immediately after it is drawn to slow the exchange of gases and altering of results. It is very critical to know both how to treat the patient and how to handle the specimen to obtain the most accurate specimen possible.

There are two hazards of arterial blood collection. Because of the higher pressure of arterial blood than venous blood, a hematoma is more likely. The arteries contain elastic tissue and provide a better closure of the puncture site for young to middle-age adults. For these adults, a hematoma is less likely. The older adult has a decrease in elastic tissue and therefore an increase in the possibility of hematoma. A patient on anticoagulant therapy has an even greater chance of a hematoma.

The second hazard is the possibility of **arteriospasm**, a reflex condition of the artery in response to pain or to anxiety. It goes away rapidly but may make it impossible to obtain blood.

There are several sites from which an accurate arterial sample can be obtained. A newborn infant during the first 24–48 hours of life has large umbilical arteries. A sick infant's respiratory system must be monitored frequently by the measurement of arterial blood gases. This measurement is completed by catheterization of the umbilical arteries. Without catheterization the umbilical arteries constrict rapidly after birth and access by needle is impossible. Shortly after birth the umbilical arteries are catheterized if the infant is premature or ill. Sampling from the catheterized artery is a duty of the infant's physician or nurse.

The preferred puncture site in adults is the radial artery located in the wrist (Figure 4.10). It is easy to palpate, and the patient is less hesitant about a puncture there. The arm and wrist of the apprehensive patient can be held more firmly to prevent movement during sample collection. The artery is also easier to compress due to the underlying bone structure after arterial puncture, making hematoma formation less likely. Collateral circulation by the ulnar artery must be checked by use of the Allen test before puncture is made in the radial artery.

The Allen test is performed by having the patient rest his or her hand on the bed or bedside table with the wrist up. The patient then clenches the fist (Figure 4.11). Using the middle and index finger of each hand, press on the radial and ulnar arteries (Figure 4.12). While continuing to hold pressure, have the patient unclench the fist (Figure 4.13). The obstructed blood flow causes a blanching of the palm. The palm and fingers should turn pink in about fifteen seconds after releasing pressure only on the ulnar artery (Figure 4.14). This indicates the ulnar artery is providing circulation to the hand and is refilling the capillary bed. In a negative test, the hand

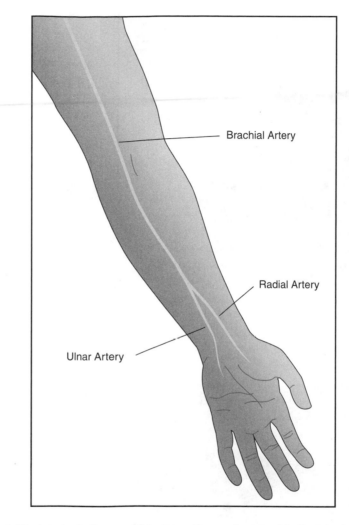

Figure 4.10 *Arteries in the arm. Note. From* Comprehensive Medical Assisting, Administrative and Clinical Competencies *(p. 824), by W. Lindh, M S. Pooler, D. C. Tamparo, and J. U. Cerrato, 1998, Albany, NY: Delmar Publishers. Copyright 1998 by Delmar Publishers. Reprinted with permission.*

remains blanched, indicating restricted blood flow of the ulnar artery. With a negative test the radial artery of that wrist should not be used and the opposite wrist should be checked.

The brachial artery can be used for arterial punctures but has several disadvantages. Its location deep within the muscles and connective tissues make palpating and puncture difficult. Once puncture is completed it is difficult to compress and stop the bleeding. Therefore hematoma formation is likely.

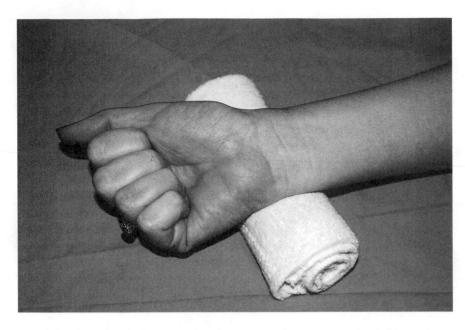

Figure 4.11 *Rest the patient's arm with the wrist up. Have patient clench fist.*

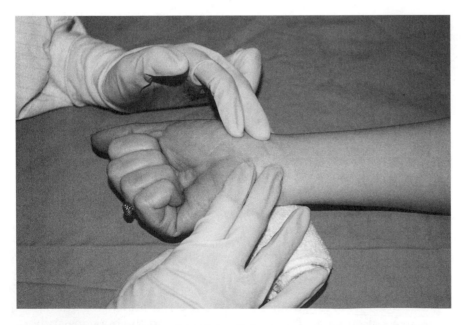

Figure 4.12 *Apply pressure to the radial and ulnar arteries simultaneously.*

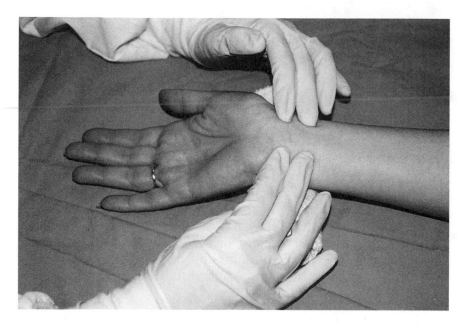

Figure 4.13 *Have the patient unclench fist.*

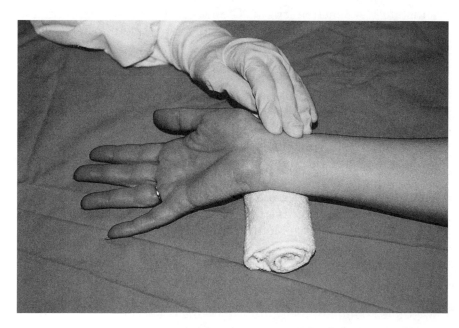

Figure 4.14 *Release pressure on the ulnar artery. Patient's hand should turn pink.*

The femoral artery is one of the largest arteries in the body. It is located in the groin and can be palpated and punctured easily due to its size. Pubic hair makes cleansing difficult and can lead to infection. The femoral artery is commonly used for cardiac catheterization and is often reserved only for catheterization-type procedures. Patients are often hesitant about arterial samples drawn from the femoral area because of the need to partially disrobe for the procedure. In newborn infants the femoral vein and nerve lie very close to the femoral artery, making puncture of the femoral artery nearly impossible without also injuring the other structures. Due to the many disadvantages of the femoral artery puncture, it is one of the last choices for arterial blood gases. Puncture of the femoral artery is generally reserved for physicians.

Arterial punctures can be done with special arterial blood sampling kits or with available supplies.

The basic equipment consists of the following:

1. An antiseptic solution such as povidine-iodine (Betadine).
2. Gauze squares.
3. A heparin solution of 1,000 IU/ml.
4. Hypodermic needles varying from 20- to 25-gauge and 5/8 inch to 1 1/2 inch in length. The size and length depend on the size of sample needed and the location of puncture site.
5. Syringes can be 1–5 ml, glass or plastic.
6. Ice water solution or bag of crushed ice.

Many types of syringes are available on the market. Glass has traditionally been the preferred type of syringe because of the limited exchange of gas through the glass and the ease with which the arterial pressure fills the syringe. The plastic syringes have now become more effective with prefilled heparin and ease of filling without manual aspiration. The exchange of gas through the plastic has become less of a factor. Evacuated tubes should not be used for arterial blood sampling. The tubes alter the partial pressure of the gas in the blood sample.

A container with ice water, or a bag of crushed ice that can maintain the sample to a temperature of 1°–5°C is used to cool the blood gas sample. The container must be large enough to immerse the barrel of the syringe. This container should be available for immediate cooling of the sample after the collection.

Patients who are to have arterial blood gases drawn are either on room air or are on an enriched oxygen mixture. The patient can be breathing spontaneously or breathing through artificial ventilation. The amount of oxygen the patient is receiving and expiring must be recorded before the blood gases are drawn. The requirements of what to record vary depending on the health care center.

The site for the draw of the radial artery is located by feeling with the middle or index finger for a pulsing action. Do not use the thumb for palpating. Once the Allen test is performed and the site is located, the site can be numbed with the lidocaine solution. Clean the skin surface with an alcohol prep. Allow the alcohol to air dry. The skin is infiltrated on top of the puncture site with a few drops of anesthetic solution. If the patient is unconscious or in adult patients who are not apprehensive about the arterial puncture, the anesthetic solution may be omitted.

The blood gas syringe is prepared by introducing anticoagulant into the syringe. The heparin vial is aseptically prepared by wiping with an alcohol swab. Draw 0.5 ml of heparin into the syringe. Pull back on the plunger to wet the entire inside barrel of the syringe. Replace the needle used to draw up the heparin with the size and type needle to be used for the arterial blood sampling. Holding the syringe with the tip of the needle upward, expel all the air and fill the dead space of the syringe and needle with heparin. Carefully replace the needle sheath over the needle, being careful not to contaminate the needle.

The patient's arm should rest on a table or pillow with the palm facing up and the wrist extended to stretch the arteries and tissues. The artery is then relocated by placing the index or middle finger over the artery to palpate for its size, depth, and direction. No tourniquet is used to help locate the artery.

The arterial puncture site is cleaned using povidine-iodine (Betadine). Before using iodine, make sure the patient does not have any allergies to iodine or shellfish. Paint the skin with the solution. Work from the puncture site to the outside in concentric circles, and then let it air dry. The povidine-iodine (Betadine) is not fully effective until it has dried. The artery can no longer be touched except with sterile gloves or fingers that have also been cleaned with the povidine-iodine (Betadine).

Remove the needle cap from the prepared syringe, and hold it as you would a dart. Place your finger over the place in the artery where you want the tip of the needle to be after it has entered the artery. Puncture the skin about 5–10 mm down the length of the artery (toward the palm) from the point the finger is feeling the pulsating artery. The needle of the syringe enters the skin at a 45-degree angle. The bevel of the needle should face the direction of the blood flow (toward the elbow). This procedure places the bevel of the needle in the center of the artery exactly under the finger that is feeling the pulsating artery (Figure 4.15). When the

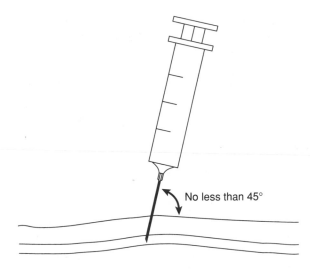

No less than 45°

Figure 4.15 *Proper position of needle entering artery.*

artery is punctured, the blood will flow into the syringe. A glass syringe will fill faster than a plastic syringe. A plastic syringe will sometimes need a slow gentle pull on the plunger. Once the syringe is filled, the needle must be removed and the syringe opening sealed with a special rubber stopper. The needle can be removed by scooping the needle sheath up with one hand and then unscrewing the needle or by using the slot on a sharps container. Do not try to bend the needle to seal off the syringe. That creates the possibility of puncturing yourself or someone else who handles the specimen. All needles must be removed from specimens before they are transported to the laboratory.

An alternate method to draw the arterial sample is to use a butterfly needle to puncture the artery. The needle of the butterfly is inserted into the artery using the same method as the syringe technique. Once the butterfly needle is in the artery, the tubing attached to the needle starts filling with blood with a pulsating action. After all the air is forced out of the tubing, a prepared heparin syringe is attached and the arterial blood obtained. The needle is removed from the patient, and the butterfly tubing is detached from the syringe and replaced with a special rubber stopper. Air must not be allowed to enter the syringe. Any air bubbles that enter the syringe must be expelled before the syringe is stopped.

Immediately after you remove the needle, place a dry gauze square over the puncture site and apply pressure for a minimum of five to ten minutes. Patients on anticoagulant blood thinners require a longer time to stop bleeding. Before you leave the patient, check that the artery has not started bleeding again.

Label the sealed specimen properly before you leave the patient's room. The sealed specimen is then completely immersed in ice water to maintain the specimen at 1°–5°C. The result of a specimen at 1°–5°C is accurate for one to two hours; at room temperature the specimen is only accurate for five to ten minutes. Waiting to immerse the specimen until after pressure is held on the patient's arm for five minutes is too long and invalidates the specimen.

An alternative to the percutaneous collection of arterial blood gases is to collect them by microcollection through skin puncture. The patient's finger or infant's foot is warmed before the puncture to obtain the maximum arterial blood flow. The capillary bed of the circulatory system is predominantly arterial blood. Blood from the microcollection must be collected in heparinized glass capillary tubes and must not contain air bubbles. Blood is collected directly into the end of the capillary tube without letting it run down the finger or foot. Exposure of the blood to air for as little as ten to thirty seconds can significantly alter the results of the blood gases. After collection, one tip of the tube is sealed with clay, a magnetic mixing bar is placed into the opposite end of the tube, and that end is then sealed with clay. The capillary tubes must then be placed on ice immediately. Due to the small size, the capillary tubes are more sensitive to temperature variation. The skin puncture blood gases are not as ideal as a percutaneous blood gas specimen. Skin puncture is necessary when removing large volumes of blood is threatening to the patient or the arteries are inaccessible. Chapter 5 covers more details of skin puncture collection.

REVIEW QUESTIONS

Multiple Choice
Choose the one best answer.

1. When drawing multiple specimens in evacuated tubes, it is important to fill which of the following color-stoppered tubes first?
   a. blue
   b. green
   c. lavender
   d. red

2. The doctor orders tests requiring a blue-top tube for coagulation studies, a lavender-top tube, a red-top tube, and a set of blood cultures. What is the correct order of draw?
   a. red, blue, blood cultures, lavender
   b. blood cultures, blue, lavender, red
   c. blood cultures, red, blue, lavender
   d. blood cultures, lavender, blue, red

3. As a general rule, you should not stick a patient more than ___ in an attempt to obtain blood.
   a. once
   b. twice
   c. three times
   d. four times

4. When you cannot perform a venipuncture successfully after two attempts, you should
   a. try at least two more times
   b. notify the patient's physician
   c. ask another phlebotomist to try
   d. request the test for the next day

5. Why is the first tube discarded when you are drawing from an indwelling arterial line?
   a. to remove tissue fluid
   b. to wipe away any bacterial contamination
   c. to remove heparin/saline contamination
   d. to make the blood flow faster

6. Which two arteries are occluded when performing the Allen's test?
   a. femoral and radial
   b. radial and ulnar
   c. brachial and ulnar
   d. radial and brachial

7. The artery that lies on the thumb side of the wrist is
   a. popliteal
   b. radial
   c. temporal
   d. ulnar

8. Pressure must be applied to the site of an arterial puncture and maintained for at least
   a. 3 minutes
   b. 5 minutes
   c. 10 minutes
   d. 15 minutes

9. In performing an arterial puncture, the artery should be punctured using a
   a. 30-degree angle of insertion with the bevel of the needle up
   b. 30-degree angle of insertion with the bevel of the needle down
   c. 45-degree angle of insertion with the bevel of the needle up
   d. 45-degree angle of insertion with the bevel of the needle down

10. An arterial puncture site is more likely to bleed than a venipuncture site because of
   a. higher blood pressure in the arteries
   b. lack of specific coagulation factors in the arteries
   c. lack of elastic tissue in the artery wall
   d. the presence of anticoagulant in the arterial syringe

Critical Thinking

1. Using your best interpersonal skills, how would you respond to a patient who says she does not want her blood drawn because all phlebotomists hurt her?

2. You have been given an order to draw patient Jane Smith in room 2232. When you go into that room, the patient identifies herself as Jane Smith but the armband indicates the patient is Jane Smiley. What do you do next?

3. The physician is in the room when you go in to draw blood, and the patient has an IV in the right forearm. The left arm is inaccessible. You need to draw a blood glucose. The physician says that you can go ahead and draw the blood in the median cubital vein of the right arm because all that is running in the IV is saline. What do you do?

4. You come back to the laboratory with a tube of blood and notice that the tube does not have a label on the tube. You have one extra label on a patient from whom you were to collect. Do you use this label to label the extra tube?

BIBLIOGRAPHY

American Association of Blood Banks. (1996). *Technical methods and procedures of the American Association of Blood Banks* (12th ed.). Philadelphia: J. B. Lippincott.

National Committee for Clinical Laboratory Standards. (1985). *Percutaneous collection of arterial blood for laboratory analysis*; Approved Standard. NCCLS Document H11-A. Villanova, PA: Author.

National Committee for Clinical Laboratory Standards. (1991). *Procedures for the collection of diagnostic blood specimens by skin puncture* (3rd ed.) Approved Standard. NCCLS Document H4-A3. Villanova, PA: Author.

National Committee for Clinical Laboratory Standards. (1998). *Procedures for the collection of diagnostic blood specimens by venipuncture* (4th ed.). Approved Standard. NCCLS Document H3-A4. Villanova, PA: Author.

Slockbower, J. M., & Blumenfeld, T. A. (1983). *Collection and handling of laboratory specimens.* Philadelphia, J. B. Lippincott.

Chapter 5

THE CHALLENGE OF PHLEBOTOMY

OBJECTIVES

After studying this chapter, you should be able to:

1. Explain the importance of communication with and reassurance of parents and child.
2. Explain the importance of proper holding techniques on children during venipuncture.
3. Explain the techniques used in venipuncture in children.
4. Describe the composition of skin puncture blood.
5. Describe skin puncture equipment.
6. State why it is important to puncture across the fingerprint line.
7. Explain the order of draw for microcollection.
8. Explain why hemolysis is more likely in skin puncture blood.
9. Explain what to do after drawing a patient receiving anticoagulant therapy.
10. Explain the best way to handle a resistant patient.
11. Describe what the phlebotomist must do before an isolation patient is drawn.

KEY TERMS

Interstitial Fluid	Fluid located between the cellular components of tissue.
Lateral	Toward the side of the body
Medial	Toward the midline, or middle, of the body.

VENIPUNCTURE ON CHILDREN

Venipuncture on children one year old and older can be an interesting challenge. Before drawing blood from a child, the phlebotomist must gain a rapport with both the child and parents. The child will not cooperate with the phlebotomist if the parent is apprehensive and does not show trust in the phlebotomist. Greet the parent and child calmly and professionally with a soft, understanding voice. Talk to the child, explaining what is going to be done. Remember this is a strange world to the child, and everything is very frightening. Children can have vivid imaginations. The phlebotomist may say blood is going to be drawn, but the child may liken the phlebotomist to the monster in a horror movie. Children should never be told the process does not hurt, but rather that it will hurt a little bit and to make it easier they need to hold still. Make this a game, and tell children they can yell as loud as they want, but just hold still. They get so involved with seeing how loud they can yell, they don't even notice the needle stick. Brace yourself for the yell.

Holding still is one of the most critical factors in obtaining an accurate blood sample from children because fighting and crying may change blood values. For the most accurate results, children must remain calm. Several people should not grab the frightened child at once. Explain to children that to make this venipuncture hurt less they must hold very still and these people are here to help them hold still. Then while you are working with the child, each person will in sequence help hold the child until everyone is holding. This leaves the child with the feeling he or she is being helped rather than ganged up on.

Limit venipuncture in children younger than two years old to superficial veins.

Successful collection of blood from superficial veins may be done with a butterfly collection set and a 23-gauge needle. Once the needle is in the vein, the flexibility of the tubing allows the child to move slightly while the blood is being collected. The butterfly also has a flash of blood in the tubing when the needle enters the vein.

Venous collection can be accomplished on children over two years old. The butterfly and the use of superficial veins are invaluable in smaller children. As the child gets older, the evacuated system is more feasible. The older child can be even more difficult to hold if the child does not want to have blood collected. If the older child can be reasoned with, the experience is not as frightening. Never underestimate how fast a child can move. Children have been known to pull the syringe out of their arm and throw it across the room. Always have someone hold the child's other hand and hold the child down.

After the venipuncture is completed, it is a good idea to offer some type of reward. A special "Best Patient" badge or cartoon bandage makes the child feel important and lets the parents know you care. The child patient requires some extra minutes to make the experience as comfortable as possible and the job easier for the next phlebotomist.

PERFORMING A SKIN PUNCTURE

The skin puncture is the method of choice in children under one year old and for adults whose veins are inaccessible. Skin puncture is done by puncturing the skin. As the patient bleeds, the blood is collected in the appropriate microcollection equipment. Adult skin punctures are done in the finger; with children under one year old, the foot is the puncture site of choice. Skin puncture of the earlobe is not recommended because the blood flow is not adequate. There are numerous limitations to this technique and only limited places the patient can be punctured safely. The blood from a skin puncture is from the capillary area of the circulatory system. This blood in the capillary bed is predominantly arterial blood. But the test result from the predominantly arterial capillary blood is generally acceptable as a substitute for venous blood.

Skin punctures in adults are used in several situations:

1. Severely burned patients.
2. Oncology patients whose veins are reserved for therapeutic purposes.
3. Obese patients where veins are too deep to locate.
4. Geriatric patients or other patients whose veins are inaccessible or very fragile.

5. Patients performing tests on themselves (home glucose monitoring).

6. Special procedures that require capillary blood (malarial smears or unopette method).

Any patients who are severely dehydrated or have poor circulation (e.g., those in shock) cannot produce a skin puncture blood sample. A patient who is extremely cold will also not produce adequate blood flow. This last situation can be rectified by the phlebotomist. The patient's hand needs to be warmed before skin puncture if there is any coolness. The best way to warm the hand is with a warm washcloth. A warm wet heat is more efficient than a dry heat or a heat pack. The washcloth should be warm to your touch as you carry it to the patient, but not so hot that it burns you. The ideal temperature is 42°C. Wrap the washcloth around the patient's hand for only three to five minutes. The washcloth will have a cooling effect due to evaporation instead of a warming effect if left on longer. The heat enlarges the capillaries, blood flows faster, and the phlebotomist obtains a better bleed. Warming of the puncture site can increase the blood flow sevenfold.

The site for the collection of a skin puncture in an adult is on the palmar surface of the distal phalanx of the finger (Figure 5.1). The side or tip of the finger should not be punctured, because the tissue is about half as thick as the tissue in the center of the finger. The fingers of choice are the middle finger and the ring finger (second and third fingers). The puncture site must be warm or have been warmed, and the finger must not be swollen from the buildup of fluids (edematous). Puncturing an edematous finger contaminates the sample with the tissue fluid. When you puncture the finger, cut across the fingerprint line. This technique delivers the best possible blood flow and facilitates the formation of drops of blood. If the cut is made between the fingerprint lines, the fingerprints exert a pressure on the cut and close the cut. Any blood that does flow follows the lines of the fingerprint, resulting in no droplet formation.

Clean the finger with isopropanol (alcohol), and then dry with a sterile gauze or allow to air dry thoroughly before any puncture. If the alcohol is not dry and contaminates the blood sample, the sample will become hemolyzed. Do not use povidone-iodine (Betadine) to clean and disinfect the puncture site. Even if the Betadine has been allowed to dry, it will cause an elevated potassium, phosphorous, or uric acid.

Puncture the finger with a lancet or with a spring-loaded lancet device. Avoid using the spring-lancet devices made for glucose monitors. These lancets produce a small round puncture and produce only two to three drops of blood, not a sufficient

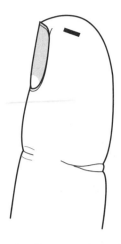

Figure 5.1 *Puncture site on finger.*

amount for most laboratory procedures. The devices that produce a small cut bleed longer and produce a sufficient amount of blood. The depth of the cut for adults varies depending on the device used. A spring-loaded device cuts to a prescribed depth. Two different principles are at work in the manufacture of spring-loaded devices. Some devices use a blade that punctures straight down with a guillotine-type action and then retracts back into the holder. The other device uses a slicing motion that produces a half-moon-type cut and then swings back into the holder. The devices that retract the blade back into the holder help associates avoid accidental punctures with contaminated devices. Some devices are gauged for the age of the fingerstick patient. The toddler device does not puncture as deeply as the adult device. With the standard lancet, the depth must also be controlled. The smaller the patient, the shallower the puncture the phlebotomist should make. One error many phlebotomists make when first doing fingersticks is to not puncture deep enough and not obtain a good bleed. Puncturing a patient's finger hurts. It is better to puncture deep enough the first time so all the blood can be obtained rather than be required to puncture more than once.

Think before the puncture. As you hold the patient's hand, position the hand so that the puncture site permits the downward flow of blood. After the puncture, the blood drips downward and gravity helps the blood flow into the collector. Before the blood sample is collected, the first drop of blood needs to be wiped away. As the finger is punctured, tissue cells are damaged, and **interstitial fluid** is released into the first drop. The subsequent drops are flowing due to arterial pressure.

If the puncture is adequate, 0.5 ml of blood can be collected from a single puncture. A drop of blood forms at the puncture site. As the drop of blood forms, touch the tip of the microcollection device to it. Blood flow can be further enhanced by gently applying continuous pressure to the surrounding tissue. Rapid milking of the finger does not enhance the blood flow. Excess pressure may cause hemolysis or contamination of the specimen with tissue fluid.

Scooping of the blood from the surface of the skin does not allow the blood to flow into the microcollection device and hemolyzes the cells. The blood will also not flow into the device when you scoop the blood, resulting in a clot before it is mixed with the anticoagulant. The microcollection device is held so the drops of blood can flow into the tip of the microcollection device and then down its walls. If blood lodges in the tip of the device, a tap of the device on a hard surface should facilitate the blood flow. Rotate the tube after every drop so the blood entering the tube contacts the anticoagulant coating the sides. Anticoagulant specimens should be mixed by inverting eight to ten times.

Figures 5.2 through 5.6 show a detailed procedure of the fingerstick of an adult using a spring-loaded lancet called a

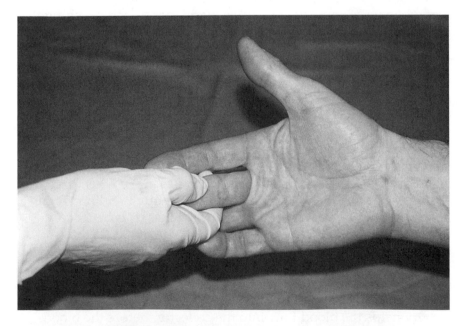

Figure 5.2 *The ambulatory patient should be seated in a standard phlebotomy chair with an arm board. This position improves fingertip blood pressure and perfusion. Supine patients should have the arm lowered to a position slightly below the breast bone. When the patient is in position, gently massage the entire length of the finger using a milking action. This increases the temperature of the finger and improves perfusion.*

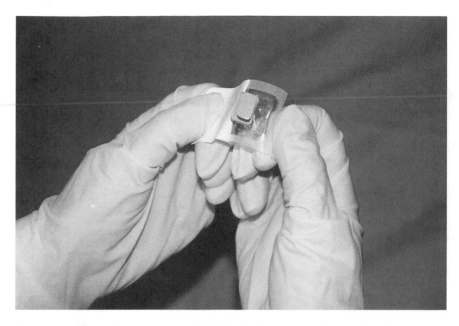

Figure 5.3 *Clean the incision site, and let it air dry. Remove the lancet from its plastic packet, taking care not to touch or contaminate the blade slot surface.*

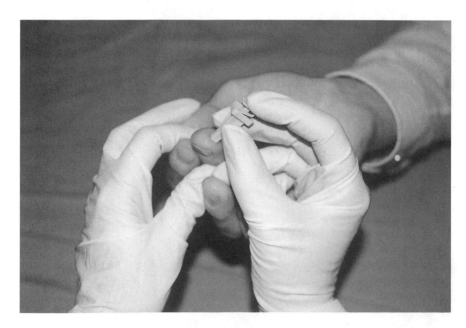

Figure 5.4 *Again massage the lower portion of the finger while avoiding the fingertip incision site. Then firmly grasp the lower portion of the finger to restrict return circulation. Firmly position the lancet device on the finger in a position to cut across the fingerprint lines. Depress the plunger with your index finger to make the puncture. Immediately release the plunger while holding the lancet on the site.*

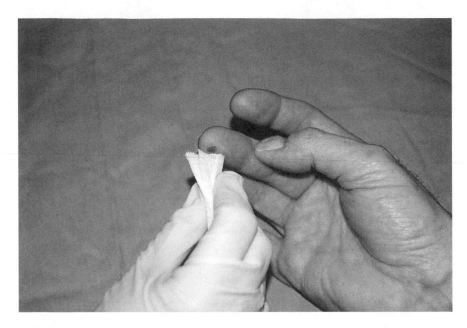

Figure 5.5 *After puncturing the finger, remove the lancet from the patient's finger. Using a gauze pad, gently wipe away the first droplet of blood. Gentle, continuous pressure on the finger ensures a free flow of blood.*

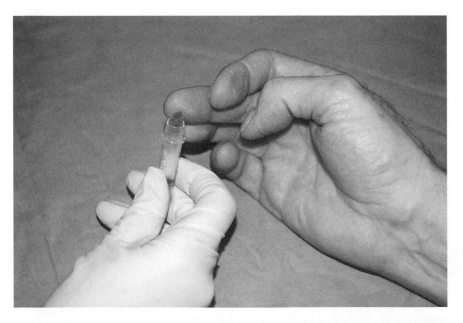

Figure 5.6 *Taking care not to make direct contact between the incision and the collection container, fill to the desired volume. Following collection, gently press a dry gauze pad to the incision.*

Microtainer lancet, manufactured by the Becton Dickinson Company. The written procedure for a fingerstick skin puncture is as follows:

PROCEDURE 5.1

FINGERSTICK SKIN PUNCTURE

Principle:

To obtain capillary blood acceptable for laboratory testing as requested by a physician.

Specimen:

Capillary blood volume dependent on the test(s).

Materials:

1. Disposable sterile lancet
2. Sterile gauze squares
3. Alcohol swabs
4. Gloves
5. Collection containers, as required by test(s).
    a. Capillary tubes
    b. Diluting fluids
    c. Calibrated pipettes
    d. Microcollection containers
6. Biohazard sharps container
7. Safety glasses and mask

Procedure:

1. Apply gloves before any patient contact.
2. Identify patient. *Inpatient*: Verify wristband name and hospital number with computer label or requisition information. *Outpatient*: Ask patient his or her name, and verify with computer label or requisition information.
3. Verify collection orders.
4. Choose finger for the puncture site that is not cold or edematous.
5. If all fingers are cold, warm the hand three minutes with a warm washcloth.

continues

PROCEDURE 5.1   *continued*

6. Select the appropriate containers for blood collection.
7. Clean the puncture site with alcohol, and let the area dry.
8. Puncture the skin with the disposable lancet. Dispose of the lancet in a sharps container.
9. Wipe away the first drop of blood with a sterile dry gauze.
10. Collect the specimen in the chosen container. Touch only the tip of the collection tube to the drop of blood. Blood flow is encouraged if the puncture site is held in a downward angle and a gentle pressure applied to the finger.
11. Seal the specimen container.
12. Anticoagulant specimens should be mixed eight to ten times.
13. Apply a bandage to the puncture site. Don't use a bandage on infants and small children, because they could swallow it and choke.
14. Label the collection containers.
15. If insufficient sample has been obtained, the puncture may be repeated at a different site. A new sterile lancet must be used, and steps 2 through 12 must be repeated.

OBTAINING A BLOOD SAMPLE ON BABIES

Obtaining a blood microcollection sample on children under one year old parallels many of the same procedures as a fingerstick sample. The one main difference is the puncture site. On infants and young children, the heel is the puncture site of choice. If an infant's heel is to be punctured, the site should be on the plantar surface **medial** to a line drawn posteriorly from the middle of the great toe to the heel, or **lateral** to a line drawn posteriorly from between the fourth and fifth toes to the heel (Figure 5.7). In almost all infants the bones, arteries, and nerves are not near these areas. On the inside (medial, or big toe side) of the heel is the posterior tibial artery (Figure 5.8) near the curvature of the heel. The outside of the heel (lateral, or little toe side) is the area that is often suggested for use to avoid possible damage to the posterior tibial artery. This caution is unwarranted when the proper incision device is used. The controlled depth of puncture devices that are commonly used eliminate this concern. The puncture should not be done in a previous puncture site, because of the possibility of infection. Do not do punctures in the central arch area of the foot. Puncture in this area may result in damage to nerves, tendons, and cartilage and offers no advantage over a heel puncture.

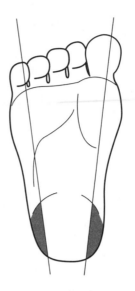

Figure 5.7 *Infant heel. The darkened areas illustrate the acceptable areas for puncture. The little toe side is the primary area of choice.*

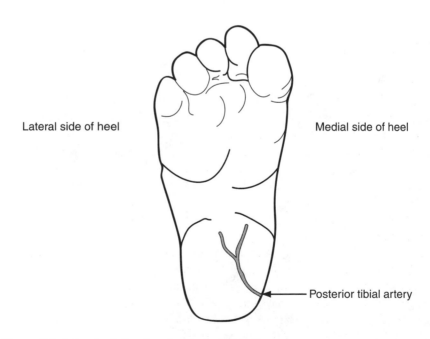

Lateral side of heel

Medial side of heel

Posterior tibial artery

Figure 5.8 *Infant heel, location of posterior tibial artery.*

The optimal depth of skin puncture from which an adequate blood sample can be obtained without injury to the infant is 2.4 mm. The capillary bed of the infant is 0.35–1.6 mm beneath the skin surface. A puncture of the plantar surface of the heel to a depth of 2.4 mm punctures the major capillary beds and does not injure the bone or nerves of the heel. Numerous devices are available commercially that meet the requirement of a puncture or 2.4 mm deep of less (see Chapter 3, "Microcollection Equipment").

Avoid puncture of the infant's fingers. The distance to the bones and main nerves of the infant's fingers is 1.2–2.2 mm. Most lancets are longer than this, and puncture of the infant's finger could result in damage to the bone or nerves with subsequent infection or permanent physical damage. The infant's finger also does not produce an adequate blood specimen.

Excessive crying of the infant can result in elevated leukocyte counts. The leukocyte count does not return to normal for up to sixty minutes. An infant who has had a procedure completed, such as circumcision, needs at least sixty minutes after crying for a blood sample to be accurate.

The procedure for microcollection from an infant is similar to a fingerstick on an adult or child. Figures 5.9–5.13 show a detailed

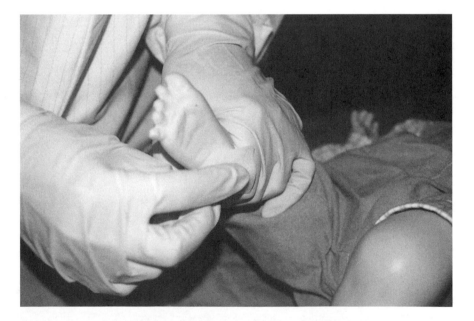

Figure 5.9 *Clean the incision area with an alcohol pad. Allow the alcohol to air dry. Do not touch the incision site or allow the heel to come in contact with any nonsterile item or surface.*

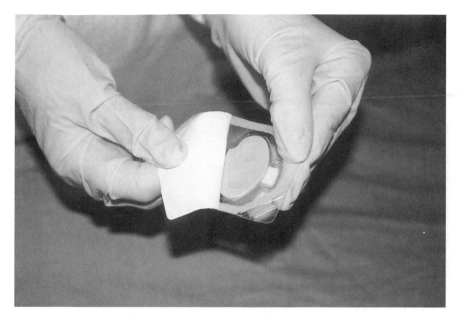

Figure 5.10 *Remove the lancet device from the package, taking care not to rest the blade end on any nonsterile surface.*

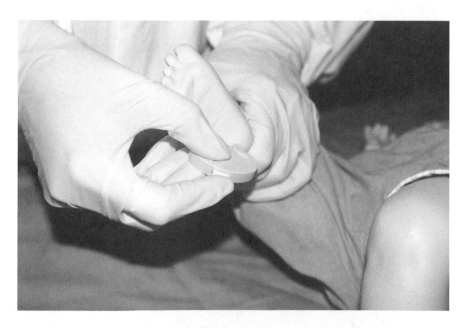

Figure 5.11 *Raise the foot above the baby's heart level, and carefully select the incision site. With gloved hand, place the blade slot area in contact with the incision area. While maintaining contact of the device with the skin, but not applying pressure, depress the plunger.*

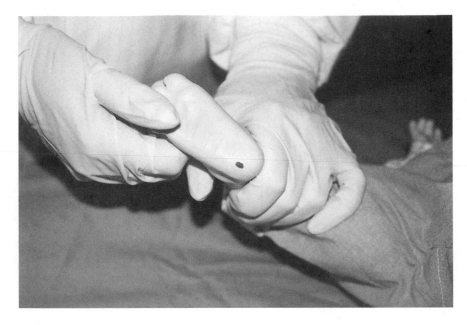

Figure 5.12 *After triggering, remove the lancet, discarding it in a sharps container. Using a dry gauze, gently wipe away the first drop of blood.*

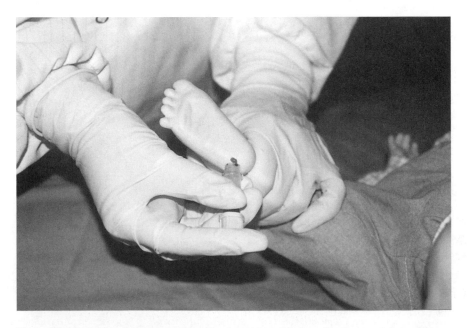

Figure 5.13 *Taking care not to make direct contact with the collection container, fill to the desired level. Following collection, press a clean dry gauze to the incision.*

procedure of the heelstick of an infant using a spring-loaded lancet called a Quick Heel manufactured by the Becton Dickinson Company. The written procedure using the infant's foot is as follows:

PROCEDURE 5.2

HEELSTICK SKIN PUNCTURE

Principle:

To obtain capillary blood acceptable for laboratory testing as requested by a physician.

Specimen:

Capillary blood volume dependent on the test(s).

Materials:

1. Disposable sterile lancet with a blade 2.4 mm long or less
2. Sterile gauze squares
3. Alcohol swabs
4. Gloves
5. Collection containers, as required by test(s)
   a. Capillary tubes
   b. Diluting fluids
   c. Calibrated pipettes
   d. Microcollection containers
6. Biohazard sharps container
7. Safety glasses and mask

Procedure:

1. Apply gloves before any patient contact.
2. Identify patient. *Inpatient*: Verify wristband name and hospital number with computer label or requisition information. *Outpatient*: Ask patient's name from the person bringing the infant in for testing and verify with computer label or requisition information.
3. Verify collection orders.
4. Choose the heel for the puncture site that is not cold or edematous.
5. Warm the foot three minutes with a warm washcloth or heel warmer.

continues

PROCEDURE 5.2   *continued*

6. Select the appropriate containers for blood collection.
7. Clean the puncture site with alcohol, and let the area dry.
8. Puncture the heel with the disposable lancet. Dispose of the lancet in a sharps container.
9. Wipe away the first drop of blood with a sterile dry gauze.
10. Collect the specimen in the chosen container. Touch only the tip of the collection tube to the drop of blood. Blood flow is encouraged if the puncture site is held in a downward angle and a gentle pressure applied to the foot.
11. Seal the specimen container.
12. Anticoagulant specimens should be mixed eight to ten times.
13. Apply a bandage to the puncture site.
14. Label the collection containers.
15. If an insufficient sample has been obtained, the puncture may be repeated at a different site. A new sterile lancet must be used and steps 2–12 must be repeated.

Several precautions must be observed to produce the most accurate specimen. Hemolysis is the greatest concern with micro-collection samples. Hemolysis may occur because of the following situations:

1. The alcohol used to clean the skin was not allowed to dry.
2. The finger or heel was squeezed to produce a greater blood flow.
3. Newborn infants have increased red blood cell fragility and a high red blood cell volume. These factors result in a higher amount of hemolysis.
4. Instead of allowing the blood to flow into the microcollection container, the blood was scraped off the skin surface.

Hemolysis as measured by the concentration of free hemoglobin in the serum or plasma of the blood may not be readily apparent. This is particularly the case in newborns with elevated bilirubins. The yellow color of the serum may mask hemolysis. Hemolyzed samples also change the concentration of chemical constituents in the blood. Potassium is elevated in all hemolyzed samples.

No known clinically important difference exists in concentration of chemical constituent between serum and heparinized plasma collected by skin puncture. When the concentrations of chemical constituents in serum or plasma from skin puncture blood are compared to those from venous blood, there does seem to be a slight statistical difference. The concentrations of glucose, potassium, total protein, and calcium have been reported to be different. Except for glucose, the concentration of those analytes is lower in skin puncture blood.

When collecting sequential samples of glucose, potassium, total protein, or calcium, the phlebotomist should use the same collection method throughout the consecutive collections. This is most significant when a series of glucose tests are collected at timed intervals, as is done in a glucose tolerance test (Chapter 6). Once a method of collection is chosen for the test, the same method should be used throughout the entire procedure to avoid variation in the results.

Producing a specimen without clots is also a challenge in microcollection. The body turns on its defenses to clot the blood at the puncture site and stop the bleeding as soon as the skin is punctured. These defenses create problems when a whole blood sample is needed. If an ethylenediamine tetraacetic acid (EDTA) specimen is required, the EDTA specimen is drawn first to obtain an adequate volume before the blood starts to clot. Any other additive specimens are collected next and clotted specimens last. If the blood has started to produce microscopic clots while filling the last tube, it is not a problem, because the blood is going to be allowed to clot in the tube.

THE ANTICOAGULATED PATIENT

The patient receiving anticoagulant therapy presents a special challenge to the phlebotomist. The patient who has been receiving anticoagulants to thin the blood is susceptible to continued bleeding and hematomas. The continued bleeding tendency should be treated after venipuncture by holding pressure on the site for at least five minutes. After the five minutes, a 2-by-2-inch gauze pad should be folded down the middle and then folded down the middle again to make a thick 1-inch square. This gauze square now has a spring to it as it tries to unfold itself. It is taped over the puncture site to produce a pressure dressing to the venipuncture site. After this is done, the patient's nurse should be asked to check the arm in fifteen minutes to check for any bleeding through the gauze. Do not allow an outpatient to leave until waiting fifteen minutes to determine if the bleeding has stopped. Remind the outpatient with a purse to carry it with the opposite arm so the puncture site does not break loose and start bleeding again.

A patient who immediately bleeds through the gauze square should have several layers of gauze placed over the site and the arm wrapped with an elastic bandage. The nurse must be asked to monitor the patient further.

Anticoagulant therapy also causes patients to develop hematomas from the venipuncture. Bleeding can often be stopped, but a hematoma still forms. This presents a problem for the next phlebotomist who has to draw blood from the patient and needs to avoid the hematoma. Sites rapidly become limited. The only way to check this tendency is to treat each anticoagulant patient as if he or she has the tendency to continue bleeding. Apply pressure to the site for five minutes and then apply a gauze pressure dressing.

THE RESISTANT PATIENT

The resistant patient can be a patient who is aware of his or her behavior and simply does not want blood drawn. The resistant patient can also be one who is semiconscious or comatose and is unaware of his or her actions. The patient who is aware does have the right to refuse to be drawn. In this case the doctor must be notified to convince the patient that the blood work is essential to the patient's recovery. Often, by taking a little time and talking to patients, you can convince them the testing is necessary, and you can overcome their resistance.

The patient who is unaware can be drawn, but the phlebotomist will need assistance in holding the patient still. Have the patient's nurse present so it can be documented in the patient's chart that the patient was held to draw the requested blood sample but not injured in the process. The phlebotomist must take special care to anticipate the patient's moves or jerks while the needle is in the arm. Gauze should be readily available, and you should be ready to release the tourniquet if the patient moves and the needle pulls out of the arm. If the needle accidentally goes much deeper, the patient's physician may need to examine the area for possible damage. If the patient is too aggressive to hold, then the physician may prescribe a sedative.

Injury to the phlebotomist, those assisting the phlebotomist, or injury to the patient must be avoided. Always remember that the patient is the customer, and the patient's wishes and legal rights must be honored.

THE PSYCHIATRIC PATIENT

The psychiatric patient often does not understand what is being done. When drawing blood from patients in a psychiatric area, the patient's nurse needs to be informed. The nurse often accompanies the phlebotomist to the patient's room to help explain the procedure to the patient or to help hold. The psychiatric patient can be unpredictable. As with the resistant patient, be ready for movement or jerks. Some patients may be suicidal. Watch your equipment to prevent patients from taking items they could use to harm themselves or someone else.

THE OBESE PATIENT

The obese patient's veins are often difficult to feel through the layers of tissue. The tourniquet has to be rather tight to exert pressure deep enough to slow the flow of venous blood. Before a venipuncture is attempted, follow the course of the vein. Obese patients have localized tissue globules under their skin that resemble veins when first feeling them, but these "veins" do not continue and will not result in blood return. The median cubital vein is usually the most prominent vein to feel. If the median cubital vein cannot be found, the veins in the hand and wrist should be more readily accessible.

THE PATIENT IN ISOLATION

No matter how many patients are drawn a day, the phlebotomist still is often hesitant to go into an isolation room and be exposed to an infection. This fear decreases with experience and knowledge of the isolation procedures that are used to protect the associate and the patient (see Chapter 2). The patient in isolation is also a challenge because of the extra protection the phlebotomist must wear while drawing the patient. This extra protection makes the job slower but safer. The protection is for the benefit of the phlebotomist and the patient.

THE PATIENT WITH DAMAGED OR COLLAPSING VEINS

Obtaining a blood sample from a patient can be challenging because of the condition of the patient's veins. The veins can be damaged and healed improperly. This is usually the result of the patient having been burned, scars on the veins through drug abuse or accidents, or surgical procedures in the areas of the veins. The damage makes the veins inaccessible because the scar tissue is too thick or the vein no longer carries blood.

A collapsing vein is weak, and the vacuum of the syringe or evacuated tube sucks the walls of the vein together so no blood can flow. The vein refills the instant the vacuum is discontinued. A syringe is the best method to obtain blood from a collapsing vein. The syringe plunger is pulled gently, a small pull at a time. The timing between the pulls allows the vein to refill. During each pull on the syringe, a small amount of blood enters the syringe. Do not work so slowly that the blood starts to clot in the syringe.

An evacuated system works to draw from a collapsing vein, but only small tubes can be used. The larger the evacuated tube, the more vacuum in the tube. If a 15-ml tube collapses the vein, instead draw five 3-ml tubes to obtain the same volume.

REVIEW QUESTIONS

Multiple Choice

Choose the one best answer.

1. The depth of the cut made by a lancet for a heel puncture must be no deeper than
   a. 3 mm
   b. 2.8 mm
   c. 2.4 mm
   d. 1.5 mm

2. The safe area for heel punctures in an infant is
   a. the arch of the foot
   b. the curvature of the heel
   c. the most medial or lateral portion of the plantar surface
   d. through previous puncture sites

3. Why must the first drop of blood from a capillary puncture be wiped away?
   a. to remove interstitial fluid
   b. to wipe away any bacterial contamination
   c. to remove heparin contamination
   d. to make the blood flow faster

4. Warming of the skin puncture site
   a. increases the blood flow through the arterioles and capillaries sevenfold
   b. results in hemolysis of the blood sample
   c. should be performed with a hot towel (60°C)
   d. should not be done routinely, because it could alter the chemical values in the blood

5. Skin puncture blood is more likely to be contaminated by
   a. hemoconcentration
   b. glycolysis
   c. hematoma
   d. hemolysis

6. If the blood is drawn too quickly from a small vein, the vein has a tendency to
   a. bruise
   b. collapse

c. disintegrate

d. roll

7. The following items are essential information for specimen labeling:

   a. the patient's complete name, the identification number, date and time the specimen was obtained, and the name of the physician

   b. the patient's complete name, the identification number, date and time the specimen was obtained, and the collector's initials

   c. the patient's complete name and the identification number

   d. the patient's complete name and the date and time the specimen was obtained

8. A conscious patient does not have an identification armband. The name and room number on the door agree with the information on the request. What should the phlebotomist do?

   a. ask the patient for verbal verification of his or her name

   b. draw the patient and take the specimen to the lab

   c. do not draw the patient until an armband has been applied

   d. draw the patient and then ask the nurse to identify the patient

9. A phlebotomist is requested to draw an unconscious patient. The room number and the name on the door agree with the request form and the patient identification armband. What else should be done to ensure patient identification?

   a. attempt to awaken the patient for verbal verification of identity

   b. attempt to find the patient's name on some other item in the room

   c. nothing else is necessary

   d. verification from a relative or a nurse of the patient's identity

10. An unconscious, unidentified man is admitted to an emergency trauma center. What would be the system of choice to ensure patient identification?

    a. assign a name to the patient, such as John Doe, and use that name for identification

    b. assign a number to the patient until the patient can be identified

    c. wait to process any samples until the patient can be identified

    d. use a three-part identification system that utilizes a temporary armband and labels for specimens and blood to be transfused

Critical Thinking

1. You open a cleaning pad and clean an infant's heel to do a heelstick, and realize that you have just cleaned it with a Betadine solution and not alcohol. What will be the result if a blood sample is collected?

2. The proper procedure is to wipe away the first drop of blood when doing a finger or heel puncture. What is the effect on the test results if the first drop is used?

BIBLIOGRAPHY

Blumenfeld, T. A., Turi, G. K.,& Blanc, W. A. (1979). Recommended site and depth of newborn heel skin punctures based on anatomical measurements and histopathology. *Lancet, 1*, 230–233.

National Committee for Clinical Laboratory Standards. (1991). *Procedures for the collection of diagnostic blood specimens by skin puncture* (3rd ed.). Approved Standard. NCCLS Document H4-A3. Villanova, PA: Author.

National Committee for Clinical Laboratory Standards. (1992, July). *Blood collection on filter paper for neonatal screening programs* (2nd ed.). Approved Standard. NCCLS Document LA4-A2. Villanova, PA: Author.

National Committee for Clinical Laboratory Standards. (1998). *Procedures for the collection of diagnostic blood specimens by venipuncture* (4th ed.). Approved Standard. NCCLS Document H3-A4. Villanova, PA: Author.

Renner, B. C., Meites, S., & Hayes, J. R. (1990). "Optimal sites and depths for skin puncture of infants and children as assessed from anatomical measurements." *Clinical Chemistry, 3*, 547–549.

Slockbower, J. M., & Blumenfeld, T. A. (1983). *Collection and handling of laboratory specimens.* Philadelphia: J. B. Lippincott.

Chapter 6

SPECIMEN CONSIDERATIONS AND SPECIAL PROCEDURES

O B J E C T I V E S

After studying this chapter, you should be able to:

1. Explain the importance of a fasting specimen.
2. Explain the importance of a timed specimen.
3. Explain the importance of specimen drawing in drug therapy monitoring.
4. Describe how a stat specimen should be handled.
5. Describe the proper procedure for making a blood smear.
6. List the characteristics of a good slide.
7. Explain the procedure of a glucose tolerance test and the two variations in how the glucose drink is administered.
8. Describe the correct procedure for a bleeding time test.
9. Explain why a bleeding time test would be performed.
10. Explain the importance of proper skin antisepsis in blood culture collection.

11. List at least four factors that will affect laboratory test values.
12. Describe the specimen collection and handling procedures for urinalysis specimens.
13. Describe proper collection procedure for semen specimens.
14. Describe proper procedure for throat culture.
15. Describe precautions necessary in transportation of specimens.

K E Y   T E R M S

Diurnal	Daily occurrence at a particular time of day.
Etiologic Agent	Viable microorganism or its toxin that causes or may cause human disease.
Fasting	Having had nothing to eat for at least 8–12 hours.
Gestational Diabetes	Diabetes during pregnancy.
Keloid	A fibrous tumor arising from a cut resulting in excessive scar tissue.
Lysis	The process of cell destruction resulting in non-intact cell structure.
NPO	Nothing by mouth. From the Latin term *non per os.*
Peak Level (Postdose)	A drug level in the blood collected 15–30 minutes after the dosage has been administered or when the highest serum concentration of the drug is expected.
Postprandial	After a meal.
Septicemia	A condition when microorganisms (mainly bacteria) are circulating and multiplying in the patient's blood.
Therapeutic Drug Monitoring (TDM)	Collection and testing of blood to evaluate and manage medication therapy effectively and safely.
Therapeutic Range	Concentration of medication that is effective and not toxic in client management.
Trough Level (Predose)	A drug level of the blood collected when the lowest serum concentration is expected, which is usually immediately before administrating the next dose.

FASTING SPECIMENS

Some tests are collected while the patient is **fasting.** A fasting specimen is collected from a patient in the morning before the patient has had breakfast and before any activities. There will often be a sign on the patient's door stating "**NPO.**" This indicates that the patient should not be given anything to eat or drink. In addition to a patient fasting to ensure accurate test results, some tests require diet restrictions. No alcohol for a number of hours before the test or a limit on certain foods are some of the restrictions. Some foods or drinks can mask the results the physician is looking for.

After the blood is drawn on a patient with restrictions, the patient may be released from the restrictions. The patient's nurse needs to be informed that you have just drawn the patient for the fasting blood work so the nurse can release the restrictions. Do not give hospital patients food or tell them they can eat without first checking with the nurse. The fasting test you just drew may be only one of several tests for which the patient must remain fasting. The patient may be going to surgery or radiology and may be fasting for those areas. The outpatient who has only come in for blood tests may be released from restrictions once you obtain the specimen.

TIMED SPECIMENS

Some specimens must be drawn at timed intervals because of medication and/or biological rhythms. These specimens should be collected at the precise time intervals required. The phlebotomist must have specific directions how the specimen should be collected and at what intervals. Tests that exhibit a **diurnal** effect are serum iron, corticosteriods, and other hormones. These are often drawn twelve hours apart in the early morning and evening.

Monitoring of a patient's drug therapy also requires a timed specimen. Aminoglycosides, coagulation therapy monitoring, digoxin, and other types of drugs are monitored at a particular time of day or a time interval after the dose of drug. All of these are monitored through **therapeutic drug monitoring (TDM).** The goal of TDM is to provide information that will allow the dose given to the patient to be effective but not toxic. This is the **therapeutic range** (Figure 6.1) for that particular drug.

Every patient will have a different metabolic rate for each drug given. The method of administration of the drug will also effect the

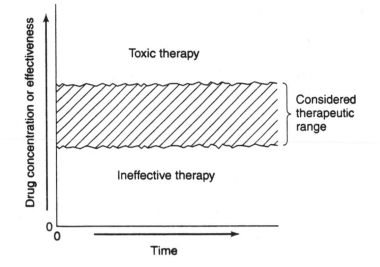

Figure 6.1 *Therapeutic range in therapeutic drug monitoring (TDM).*

metabolism of the drug. The drug may be given orally or injected intramuscularly or intravenously. The timing of collection of the specimens is critical to the proper determination of the level of drug in the patient. Many variables influence the effectiveness of the drug:

1. Drug half-life.
2. Concentration of medication.
3. Form of drug administration.
4. Age of the patient.
5. Weight of the patient.
6. Liver function.
7. Kidney function.
8. Disease state.
9. Interacting drug therapy.
10. Patient's metabolism.

Levels for drugs are collected to determine how effectively the drug is working. Since each patient varies in how he or she responds to the drug, each patient must be tested. The patient is tested for a prespecimen before the drug is given and then for a postspecimen after the drug has been administered.

The prespecimen drawn when the drug is at the lowest level in the patient is known as the **trough level (predose).** The trough is

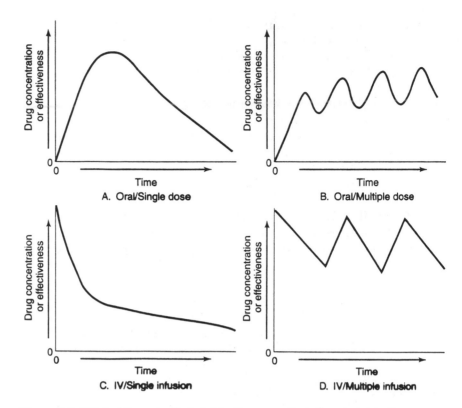

Figure 6.2 *Effect of the route of administration verses time after administration.*

usually drawn five minutes before the drug is administered. The drug is usually administered through an intravenous (IV) injection. Once the drug has been completely administered for a specific period of time, the **peak level (postdose)** is collected. This peak level should be collected at a time the drug is at its highest level in the patient. This peak level should fall somewhere in the therapeutic range. The patient's response time to the therapy depends on the method of administration. With an oral medication, the peak will not occur for a period of time. The level will then drop rapidly until another dose is given. The impact with an IV is almost immediate and then also diminishes rather quickly. (Figure 6.2). The following example illustrates the proper timing.

Pre- and Postserum Levels

Aminoglycosides (amikacin, gentamicin, tobramycin)
   Predose five minutes before infusion.
   Postdose five minutes after 30-minute infusion.

Example: Pre and post aminoglycoside with 10:00 A.M. dose.
            Predose drawn at   9:55 A.M.
            Dose infused at   10–10:30 A.M.
            Postdose drawn at   10:35 A.M.

Vancomycin
    Predose five minutes before infusion.
    Postdose one hour after a one-hour infusion.
    Example: Pre- and postdose vancomycin levels with 10 A.M. dose.
                Predose drawn at   9:55 A.M.
                Dose infused at   10–11:00 A.M.
                Postdose drawn at   12 noon

These examples give the ideal timing of the draws. In reality, the phlebotomist is not able to draw the patient at precisely the moment requested. Because of travel time to the patient and other patients to draw, the draw times may be off by ten to fifteen minutes. This is not critical as long as the exact time of the draw is documented. From the draw times and the amount of drug level in the patient, the pharmacist calculates the next dose size the patient should receive. Most hospitals require documenting the exact time the specimen was drawn both on the tube of blood and in the computer. Both of these times should match exactly.

STAT SPECIMENS

Stat specimens must have the phlebotomist's immediate attention. A true stat order is so critical that not obtaining it and processing it immediately could lead to the death of the patient. The stat is one of the most variable orders. Many tests are ordered stat for a true stat need. Often the stat is not ordered for emergency reasons. Reasons can vary. For example, the physician may need the results before the patient is sent home, or someone forgot to order the test and the physician is coming in to make rounds.

Because the criticalness of the stat varies, some hospitals have instituted different levels of the stat test, or a middle of the road priority such as ASAP (as soon as possible). A stat test must be handled in such a way as to obtain it and deliver it to the laboratory as fast as possible. Even if the patient does not look critical, the specimen must be handled as ordered. All phlebotomy must be completed with all the proper steps. Never take shortcuts to speed the processing.

SPECIAL COLLECTION TECHNIQUES

Some tests require special collection techniques for the accuracy of the procedure.

Alcohol

When drawing blood for alcohol testing, use a disinfectant solution other than alcohol. Alcohol swabbing of the phlebotomy site, even when allowed to dry, contaminates the blood specimen and falsely raises the alcohol level of the patient. Solutions such as zephrin chloride, soap, or hydrogen peroxide are acceptable. Do not use Betadine or iodine swabs because these contain alcohol. Care must also be taken with these specimens because the results are often needed for legal reasons.

Chain of Custody

For chain of custody on forensic specimens, where the results will possibly be used in a court case, a special chain of custody procedure should be followed. The chain of custody procedure dictates that each person handling the specimen must sign a form. The form indicates who the person received the specimen from, who it was given to, and the length of time the person had the specimen. The specimen is also transported in a locked box to prevent the possibility of switching or tampering with it. This chain of custody guarantees the integrity of the specimen to the court.

Heavy Metals

Heavy metals is a procedure to follow when blood is being tested for heavy metals, such as arsenic or lead. These are sometimes called trace elements. The only difference in the collection is that the blood must be collected in a special metal-free tube. These are usually royal-blue-stoppered tubes that may or may not contain an anticoagulant. The glass and rubber stoppers have been specially refined to be metal free. Traces of metal in the routinely used evacuated tube may leach into the specimen and give the patient a falsely elevated heavy metal value. Microsamples collected for heavy metals require that the skin be cleansed thoroughly to avoid any contamination of the sample from residual heavy metal on the skin surface.

Therapeutic Phlebotomy

Polycythemia is a disease that causes an increase in the number of erythrocytes in a patient's blood. One method of treating the disease is through the use of therapeutic phlebotomy that draws large amounts of blood from the patient. This reduces the strain on the heart and other body systems. The amount of blood taken at one treatment is 500 ml. This is done in the same manner as if the patient was making a donation of blood to the blood bank. The blood is then discarded and not used for someone else.

MAKING A BLOOD SMEAR

Blood smears are needed for microscopic examination of the blood. They may be prepared from venous blood or from capillary blood. The most common blood smear is used for the peripheral smear used for a complete blood count (CBC) differential. Blood smears are also made for such tests as malarial smears and special hematology procedures. The blood is spread on a glass slide to produce a wedge or thin smear. A good smear has a feathered edge that is nearly square and a rainbow sheen when reflecting light. The perfect slide consists of a smear that is exactly one cell thick in the feathered edge.

The procedure for making a blood smear with a feathered edge is as follows and is pictured in Figure 6.3.

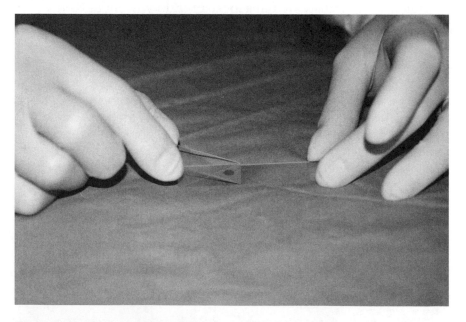

Figure 6-3A *Blood smear preparation. Rest the end of the spreader slide at a 45-degree angle just in front of the drop of blood.*

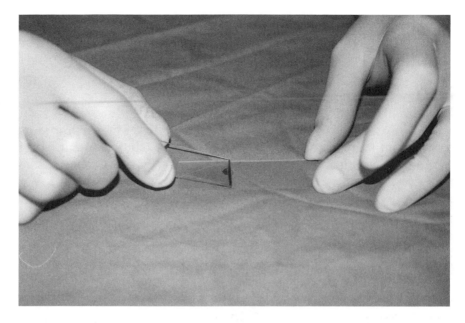

Figure 6.3B *Draw the spreader slide backward until it just touches the drop of blood.*

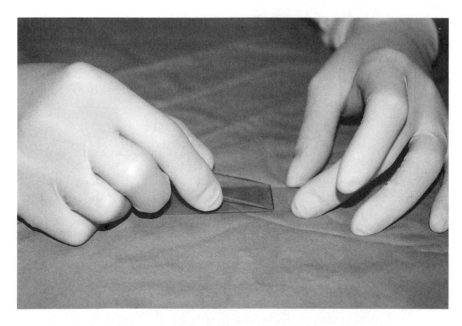

Figure 6.3C *Push the spreader slide rapidly across the stationary slide with an even stroke and pressure.*

PROCEDURE 6.1

MAKING A BLOOD SMEAR

Principle:

Properly and safely prepare a blood smear on a microscopic slide from anticoagulated or capillary blood. Prepare the blood smear, altering as little as possible the form, structure, or distribution of the cells.

Materials:

Gloves
Hand disinfectant
Capillary tubes
Materials for capillary puncture
Anticoagulated blood
70 percent alcohol
Microscope slides (1 inch by 3 inches)
Biohazard container for sharps

Procedure:

1. Wash hands or use hand disinfectant if handwashing facilities are not available.
2. Select two glass slides that are clean and free of chipped edges. Fingerprints, grease, dust, or powder from gloves on the surface of the slides will make them unacceptable. Gloves should be worn for the remaining steps of the procedure.
3. Place a drop of blood 1–2 mm in diameter on one of the slides. The drop should be in the center line approximately 1/4 inch from the frosted edge of the slide.
4. Hold the slide with the drop of blood at the opposite end with the thumb and forefinger of your nondominant hand. Grasp the spreader slide similarly with your dominant hand.
5. Rest the end of the spreader slide at a 45-degree angle just in front of the drop of blood (Figure 6.3A).
6. Draw the spreader slide backward until it just touches the drop of blood. The blood should spread to the edges of the slide. The blood must spread evenly along the interface of the two slides. Not spreading the blood evenly will cause a pointed feathered edge (Figure 6.3B).
7. Keep the spreader slide at the 45-degree angle. Push the spreader slide rapidly across the stationary slide with even stroke and pressure (Figure 6.3C). Any pressure exerted on the spreader slide should be

continues

PROCEDURE 6.1   *continued*

directed across the slide in the direction that the film is made rather than down on the stationary slide. The faster the spreader slide is moved, the longer and thinner the film will be. The slower the slide is moved, the shorter and thicker the slide will be. The angle will also vary the results. An angle greater than 45 degrees makes the smear thicker; less than 45 degrees, the smear is thinner. Speed, angle, and drop size can be varied slightly to produce a good smear.

8. Allow the slide to air dry. To facilitate air drying, fan the slide back and forth by holding between thumb and forefinger. Do not blow on the slide.

9. Check the slide for acceptability. The smear should cover approximately three-fourths of the length of the slide. The feathered edge should be relatively straight (Figure 6.4). It should have a rainbow appearance when reflecting light. The smear should be smooth the entire length of the slide with no holes or grainy appearance.

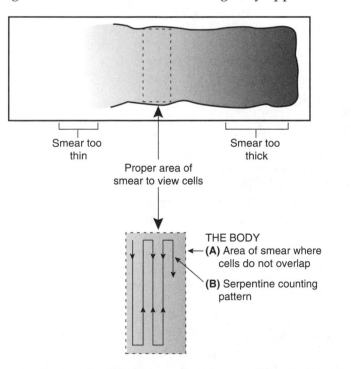

Figure 6.4 *Straight-edge (peripheral) blood smear. Proper area of slide to be viewed for differential cell count: (A) close-up of proper body and (B) counting pattern. Note. From Comprehensive Medical Assisting, Administrative and Clinical Competencies (p. 868), by W. Lindh, M. S. Pooler, D. C. Tamparo, and J. U. Cerrato, 1998, Albany, NY: Delmar Publishers. Copyright 1998 by Delmar Publishers. Reprinted with permission.*

continues

PROCEDURE 6.1 *continued*

10. Write the patient information on the slide using pencil or special marking pen. The patient information is written on the slide at the thick end of the smear. If a frosted-end slide is used, the information is written on the frosted area. The ink from ballpoint pens would wash off when the slide is processed.

It takes considerable practice to make good slides consistently. There are slide-making devices on the market. These are too large to carry with you and are designed to work with automated differential reading instruments. Some of these devices make an actual wedge smear, while others spin the slide to create a monolayer of cells over the entire slide. The handmade wedge or thin slide is the most commonly made blood film.

For malaria diagnosis, a second type of blood film, called a thick smear is also used. This is not a smear at all but consists of a large drop of blood about the size of a dime placed in the center of the slide and allowed to dry. This thick drop of blood is then visually checked for the malarial organism.

GLUCOSE TESTING

Diabetes mellitus is a complicated disease that may cause more complications for the patient than just an increased blood glucose level. Persons with diabetes mellitus often develop blindness, kidney failure, or circulatory problems that result in tissue damage and possible amputation. Hyperglycemia is the signal that a person possibly has diabetes mellitus. Commonly, the patient is deficient in insulin production by the pancreas or in insulin function. Insulin-dependent diabetes mellitus, Type I, means a person produces very little insulin or no insulin. The non-insulin-dependent diabetes mellitus, Type II, is present in 80–90 percent of diabetes patients. Most patients of this type have a normal insulin concentration but lack relative insulin activity. These patients often have fasting blood glucose levels within normal limits but are unable to metabolize ingested glucose properly. The glucose tolerance test (GTT) detects the borderline diabetic by measuring the patient's ability to dispose of a large oral intake of glucose.

A number of factors can affect glucose tolerance and should be controlled before the test is performed. When a GTT is ordered, the patient should omit medications that are known to affect a glucose tolerance, have three days of unrestricted diet, and have unrestricted activity. The test should then be performed in the morning after an eight- to sixteen-hour fast. The patient should not be allowed coffee or cigarettes and should try to keep anxiety to a minimum.

A fasting blood specimen is obtained. The glucose level of the blood is then determined. Depending on the result of the glucose analysis, one of the following courses of action should be taken. If the fasting glucose specimen is greater than 140 mg/dl, no GTT is necessary. If the fasting specimen is less than 140 mg/dl, then the GTT should be completed. The value of 140 mg/dl varies depending on the laboratory.

The patient is given a flavored drink containing 75 grams of glucose for the standard GTT. The dosage for children 12 years and under is 1.75 grams per kilogram of body weight. For a gestational GTT, the drink must contain 100 grams of glucose. The drink must be ingested within five minutes. After ingestion of the drink, the time is started.

Blood specimens are then drawn at thirty minutes, one hour, two hours, three hours, and so on, after the dose. The GTT is carried out for the length of time the physician has requested. Generally, this is three to five hours. The same type of blood specimen must be obtained for the entire test. If venous blood is collected for the fasting specimen, all specimens must be collected as venous blood. A capillary fasting specimen dictates that capillary blood be collected for the remainder of the test. Once a method of collection is chosen for the test, the same method should be used throughout the entire procedure to avoid variation in the results. Capillary blood has a slightly higher value for glucose than a venous sample taken at the same time. If a capillary sample is collected in the middle of the GTT, this value will be slightly higher than the other venous samples. Any specimens that are collected in tubes without a preservative must be centrifuged immediately to prevent glycolysis.

The criteria for diagnosis of diabetes can be based on fasting glucose concentrations or glucose tolerance values. A GTT can be used to indicate what type of diabetes is present.

Diabetes Mellitus

Diabetes mellitus is indicated by a two-hour plasma glucose concentration greater than 200 mg/dl during the GTT. At least one value between zero time and two hours registers greater than 200 mg/dl.

Questionable/Borderline Diabetes Mellitus

Questionable/borderline diabetes mellitus is indicated by a GTT result of a two-hour plasma glucose concentration greater than 140 mg/dl and less than 200 mg/dl. At least one value between zero time and two hours must be greater than 200 mg/dl.

Gestational Diabetes

Gestational diabetes is a case of diabetes that has developed during a woman's pregnancy. The diabetes must be monitored like any other diabetes but is usually controlled through regulated and monitored eating habits. This type of diabetes is usually not permanent. When the woman is no longer pregnant, her metabolism of glucose returns to her pre-pregnancy metabolism. Gestational diabetes is diagnosed when two or more of the following plasma glucose values are met or exceeded (after 100 grams of glucose dose):

Fasting	105 mg/dl
One-hour	190 mg/dl
Two-hour	165 mg/dl
Three-hour	145 mg/dl

Normal Glucose Tolerance

A glucose tolerance is considered normal if the fasting plasma glucose is less than 140 mg/dl. The two-hour glucose concentration is less than 140 mg/dl.

Hyperinsulinism

Hyperinsulinism is indicated by the GTT if the fasting glucose is less that 70 mg/dl. All glucose concentrations remain less than normal.

The values obtained in a GTT can be graphed to determine the severity of the diabetes compared to normal values (Figure 6.5).

Postprandial Glucose Test

Instead of starting with a GTT, the physician often orders a **postprandial** blood sugar drawn two hours after a meal. A normal patient's blood glucose is not elevated two hours after a meal. A diabetic patient has an elevated glucose after a meal. These are used as a screening test after a patient has shown elevated levels on a fasting blood glucose.

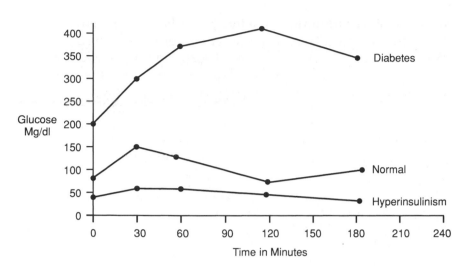

Figure 6.5 *Glucose tolerance test.*

Two-Hour Postglucose Drink

Giving a patient a glucose load as in a GTT and then testing the patient's glucose two hours later is more objective than the postprandial glucose. This method standardizes the amount of glucose given and eliminates the variables of time to consume the meal and how fast the meal is absorbed. The patient has the benefit of not being drawn as many times as with a glucose tolerance.

Home Monitoring of Glucose

Persons with diabetes do not want to go to the laboratory to be tested on a daily basis. Several instruments for home monitoring are available for patient purchase. All the instruments use the same basic principle. Patients fingerstick themselves and put a drop of blood on a small testing pad. The pad is then inserted into the instrument, and at the proper time the glucose value is read. Patients record the value and can even be trained to adjust their insulin dose depending on the glucose values.

Xylose Tolerance

All testing of patients is not done with glucose as the sugar. D-xylose is a sugar that is used in a tolerance test to determine malabsorption. D-xylose is a pentose not normally present in the blood. When given orally, it is absorbed in the small intestine, passed unchanged through the liver, and then excreted by the kidneys. The xylose tolerance test is an indication of the absorption function of the intestine. Low absorption is observed in intestinal malabsorption or in bacterial overgrowth of the intestine. Low absorption is not noted in pancreatic insufficiency.

The tolerance is conducted by giving the patient 25 grams of D-xylose dissolved in water. A two-hour blood sample is taken, and all urine excreted over five hours is collected. The amount of xylose is then determined, and the blood and urine values are compared.

BLEEDING TIMES

The bleeding time is the time it takes a standardized incision to stop bleeding. When a vessel is injured in a patient with normal coagulation function, platelets adhere to the exposed wound and lining of the vessel. Platelets then aggregate at the incision site, forming the primary platelet plug. The bleeding time is a measure of the functional integrity of the small blood vessels and the ability of platelets to form hemostatic plugs to stop bleeding. The bleeding time is prolonged in disease that affects the ability of vessels to constrict and retract and in disease in which there is a decrease in platelet number (thrombocytopenia). Diseases that decrease platelet function, such as thrombasthenia and thrombocytopathy, also increase bleeding time. Aspirin, aspirin-containing drugs, certain anticoagulants, antibiotics, and antihistamines may cause a prolonging of the bleeding time in normal patients. Any aspirin or bleeding-time-prolonging drugs should be eliminated for one week before the test.

It is important to know that the bleeding time is affected the most when the platelet count falls below 100,000 per cubic millimeter. It is good practice to have a platelet count on the patient before a bleeding time is attempted. It is fruitless to expect a bleeding time to be normal when the platelet count is decreased.

Historically there are several methods of performing the bleeding time. The Duke method is the oldest method and was performed by puncturing the earlobe with a lancet, making a 3-mm-deep incision. The Ivy method was developed later to help standardize the technique and make the procedure more sensitive.

Currently available commercial devices such as used in the Surgicutt method are a continued refinement of the Ivy method. These commercially available devices have standard-ized the bleeding time test to give more accurate, reproducible results. Several different devices are available. Devices can be purchased that make one or two incisions. What is illustrated here (Figure 6.6A–I) is a single-incision device called Surgicutt produced by the International Technidyne Corporation of Edison, New Jersey. The Surgicutt device uses an automated incision-making device to make the cut for the bleeding time. The device is spring-loaded and provides a standard cut 5 mm in length and 1 mm in depth. When triggered, the blade protracts down, sweeps across, and automatically retracts back into the device. This retracting of the blade adds a safety feature, preventing accidental cutting of the phlebotomist with a contaminated lancet.

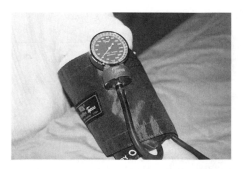

Figure 6.6A *Place the blood pressure cuff on the patient's arm. Inflate the cuff to 40 mm Hg.*

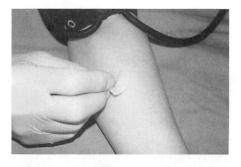

Figure 6.6B *Clean the outer surface of the patient's forearm with alcohol; allow to air dry.*

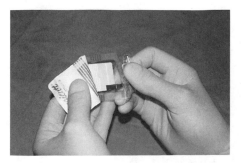

Figure 6.6C *Remove the Surgicutt device from the package, being careful not to touch the blade slot end on any nonsterile surface.*

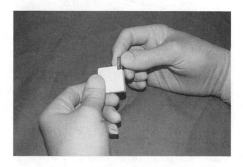

Figure 6.6D *Remove the safety clip. Do not push the trigger or touch the blade slot.*

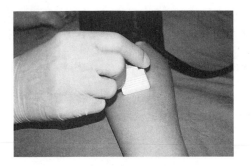

Figure 6.6E *Gently rest the device on the patient's forearm at the location away from any superficial veins. Gently push the trigger, and start the stopwatch simultaneously.*

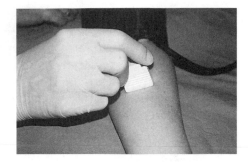

Figure 6.6F *Remove the device from the patient's forearm immediately after triggering.*

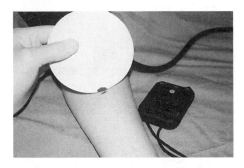

Figure 6.6G *Blot the blood with filter paper at regular thirty second intervals.*

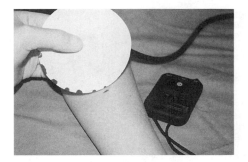

Figure 6.6H *Wick the blood every thirty seconds until no blood stains the paper. Stop the timer.*

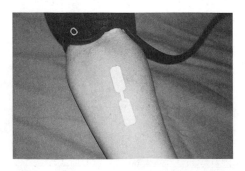

Figure 6.6I *Close the incision with a wound closure strip.*

PROCEDURE 6.2

SURGICUTT BLEEDING TIME METHOD

Principle:

The Surgicutt bleeding time test uses a standardized incision and pressure to determine the length of time a patient takes to stop bleeding. This time is indicative of possible bleeding tendencies in the patient.

Materials:

Sphygmomanometer (blood pressure cuff)
Surgicutt bleeding time device
Circle filter paper (No. 11, Whatman Inc., Clifton, NJ)
Stopwatch
Alcohol wipes
Gauze pads
Wound closure strip
Gloves

Procedure:

1. Verify patient identity.
2. Apply gloves before any patient contact.
3. Place the patient's arm on a steady support with the volar surface exposed. The incision is best performed over the lateral aspect, volar surface of the forearm, parallel to and 5 cm below the antecubital crease. Avoid surface scars, bruises, surface veins, and edematous areas.
4. Place the blood pressure cuff on the patient's upper arm. Inflate the cuff, and maintain pressure at 40 mm Hg. The time between inflation of cuff and incision should be no more than 30 seconds. Hold at this exact pressure for the duration of the test (Figure 6.6A).
5. Clean the outer surface of the patient's forearm with alcohol; allow to air dry (Figure 6.6B).
6. Remove the Surgicutt device from the pack, being careful not to contaminate the instrument by touching or resting the blade-slot end on any unsterile surface (Figure 6.6C).
7. Remove the safety clip. Do not push the trigger or touch the blade slot (Figure 6.6D).
8. Observe the patient's forearm for superficial veins. Determine a location away from any superficial veins. Gently rest the device on

continues

PROCEDURE 6.2   *continued*

the patient's forearm at the location selected, and apply minimal pressure so both ends of the device are lightly touching the skin. The incision is best performed parallel to the anticubital crease (Figure 6.6E).

9. Gently push the trigger and start the stopwatch simultaneously.

10. Remove the device from the patient's forearm immediately after triggering (Figure 6.6F).

11. Blot the blood with the filter paper at regular 30-second intervals. Do not touch the paper directly to the incision, so as not to disturb the platelet plug (Figure 6.6G).

12. Wick the blood every 30 seconds from then on until blood no longer stains the paper. Stop the timer. Bleeding time is determined to the nearest 30 seconds (Figure 6.6H).

13. Remove the blood pressure cuff, and cleanse the area with an alcohol swab. Potential scarring and **keloiding** can be reduced by closing the edges of the incision with a wound closure strip for 24 hours (Figure 6.6I). Inform the patient there will be a small scar present after healing.

14. Dispose of the bleeding time device in a sharps container.

Normals: 2–8 minutes

Comments: If the patient continues to bleed after 15 minutes, stop the test and apply pressure to the wound.

Hints on Technique:

1. The pressure placed on the Surgicutt device affects the bleeding time.

2. The incision may be made either parallel or perpendicular to the anticubital crease. Results will vary depending on the direction of the incision; therefore, one direction should be used consistently.

3. Blood should flow freely within 20 seconds.

THE BLOOD CULTURE

Blood cultures are collected whenever it is suspected that a patient has septicemia. **Septicemia** is a condition when microorganisms (mainly bacteria) circulate and multiply in the patient's blood. Since blood is normally sterile, the presence of microorganisms and their products is very serious and can cause death. The blood is collected and placed in a bottle containing a solution that enhances the growth of significant microorganisms. An anticoagulant is also present. The microorganisms can then be cultured and identified so the most effective antibiotic treatment can be started.

If blood cultures are to be collected after antimicrobial treatment has started, the blood culture must be drawn in a special bottle containing a resin solution to inactivate the antimicrobial agent. This allows the bacteria to grow. The resin bottle is known as an antibiotic removal device (ARD) bottle. Antimicrobial agents can also be inactivated by placing penicillinase (beta-lactamase) in the media after the blood cultures have been collected. Care must be taken in doing this so as not to contaminate the blood culture. A microorganism that contaminates the culture could be interpreted as coming from the patient and misdirect the physician's treatment.

The volume of blood needed is critical to optimal recovery of the microorganisms. Up to 10 ml of blood may be placed in the bottle. The optimal amount of blood varies depending on the manufacturer of the blood culture bottles. In infants and children, 1–5 ml of blood in a pediatric bottle is sufficient.

Additional amounts of blood are unlikely to increase the yield and only contribute to hospital-acquired anemia. The human serum itself is lethal to microorganisms. In most instances a 1:10 to 1:20 dilution of blood to broth is needed. For optimum yield of microorganisms, the bottles should not be overfilled or underfilled.

The blood cultures are drawn in sets of two bottles. One bottle is the aerobic bottle for those microorganisms that need oxygen to grow. The second bottle is an anaerobic bottle for the microorganisms requiring an environment without oxygen. A set of blood cultures used to be collected at the height of the patient's fever when the microorganisms were thought to be at their greatest number in the blood. With the new high-recovery blood culture bottles available, drawing of the blood at the height of the fever is not as critical. Even during a low point of the fever, the microorganisms are in sufficient number for rapid growth.

Recent reports recommend that in most instances two blood culture sets are sufficient for recovery of significant microorganisms, particularly with the increased blood volume collected. There is greater than 99 percent recovery with only two sets. Ideally, the two sets are at separate venipuncture sites before starting therapy.

The most critical step in collecting a blood culture is the proper cleansing of the site. The site must be as clean as possible to avoid contaminating the blood culture with skin surface microorganisms and producing a false-positive blood culture. The site must first be cleansed with alcohol to remove the oils and dirt on the skin surface. The site is then cleansed with a 2 percent tincture of iodine solution. The cleansing is done with a circular motion, starting at the site of the puncture and moving in concentric circles outward. The iodine is painted on the area, not flooded over the site. Iodine is an effective antiseptic only if it is allowed to dry before the venipuncture is attempted. Before any cleansing of the site is begun, the patient must be asked about any allergy to iodine. If the patient does have an iodine allergy, the only recourse is to cleanse thoroughly with 70 percent alcohol. As with most techniques, the cleansing procedure varies from one laboratory to another.

The seals on the bottles are broken off. This seal usually consists of a metal flip-off cap. Under the seal is a rubber septum through which the blood is injected. Once the flip-off cap is removed, the septum is cleansed with an alcohol pad. The alcohol pad is left on the bottle until just before the blood is injected. The proper amount of blood is then drawn with a syringe. The alcohol pad is removed from the bottle cap. Without changing needles, the phlebotomist then injects blood into the bottles. Always inject the anaerobic bottle first to maintain a strict anaerobic environment.

Instead of using a syringe to draw the blood and inoculate the bottles, the phlebotomist can use a butterfly collection set. Adapters are available that attach to the rubber-sleeved end of the butterfly (Figure 6.7). The top of each bottle is cleansed with alcohol. The patient's vein is accessed with the butterfly needle. The adapter is first slipped over the top of the aerobic bottle and then the anaerobic bottle. Once the needle punctures the bottle, the bottle begins to fill with blood. Each bottle is filled to the proper level of blood. Once the blood cultures are collected, additional tubes of blood can be drawn without drawing the patient again.

There are also blood culture bottles with long necks that insert into an evacuated needle holder. The tops of the bottles are cleansed with alcohol. The blood is drawn directly into the special bottle, and the media is directly inoculated. A standard evacuated needle and holder are used for collection. After the blood cultures are drawn, any additional tubes of blood can be drawn without a second venipuncture.

A method of indirect inoculation of the blood culture media is done by using an Isolator collection tube. The patient's arm is cleansed the standard way. The top of the tube is cleaned with alcohol. Ten milliliters of blood are drawn directly into the Isolator tube using a standard evacuated needle and holder. The tube is inverted five to six times after collection. The blood cells in the

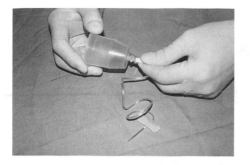

Figure 6.7A *Attach the butterfly to the adapter.*

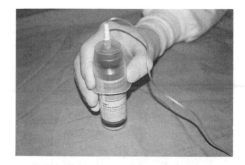

Figure 6.7B *Slide the adapter over the top of the blood culture bottle.*

tube **lyse,** the tube is centrifuged in the microbiology laboratory, and the sediment is then inoculated directly on solid culture media to determine if microorganisms are present.

With all blood culture methods, there are some variations in procedure for the phlebotomist. The arm cleansing technique may differ. Some blood culture systems must have the aerobic bottle vented (air added) by the phlebotomist. A variation in procedure does not indicate the laboratory is improper but illustrates variations in manufacturers.

FACTORS AFFECTING LABORATORY VALUES

Numerous variables can affect test results. Once some of these variables are in play, the most expensive analytical instrument on the market cannot give an accurate and precise result. Some of these factors are the responsibility of the phlebotomist, while others reflect the physiological factors of the patient. The tourniquet is a factor under the phlebotomist's control that can create a change in test results. The tourniquet should not be on the arm longer than one minute. The patient who makes an extremely tight fist or pumps the hand also changes the analyte concentration. Potassium, phosphorous, and lactate are a few of the analytes that increase with prolonged tourniquet placement or hand activity.

The phlebotomist also has control of whether or not the specimen should be collected. The phlebotomist should always ask patients if they are fasting for tests that require a fasting specimen. Some specimens must be drawn at timed intervals because of medication or diurnal rhythm. The precise timing of the specimen collection is critical. The exact time of collection must also be noted on the specimen.

An incorrect volume of blood in the tube can change results. It is best to provide the laboratory with the properly filled tube to begin with because the patient may not be readily available for a redraw. The ethylenediamine tetraacetic acid (EDTA) tube should be filled to at least 75 percent of the stated volume. Any less blood will cause a dilutional factor and causes the red blood cells to decrease in size. Too much blood in the tube causes a clotting of the blood. Citrate tubes are the most critical for correct fill size. The variation in fill can only be plus or minus 10 percent from the stated volume. Any greater variation affects test results.

Defective tubes give an improper fill even with the best venipuncture. Tubes should vary no more than plus or minus 10 percent in filling. To quality-control the tubes, use a syringe filled with water. The syringe should be filled with more water than the capacity of the tube that is being tested. The top of the tube is punctured with the syringe needle, and the amount of water the tube pulls from the syringe is noted. If several tubes vary more than 10 percent from the stated volume of the tube, the tubes are defective. Contact the manufacturer to resolve the problem.

The proper heparin tube to use can be confusing for even the most experienced phlebotomist. Ammonium, lithium, and sodium heparin are all available for use. Certain tests are affected by using the wrong heparin tube. Testing for sodium from a sodium heparin tube can elevate the patient's sodium value. In the same manner, lithium is increased in a lithium heparin tube. Chromosome studies need sodium heparin because lithium is toxic to cells. If a heparin tube is to be drawn, check that the correct type of heparin tube is used.

The order of draw is the most abused factor that varies test results over which the phlebotomist has control (see Chapter 4). Blood must be collected with the patient's arm in the arm-down position to prevent the anticoagulated blood from flowing back into the needle and contaminating the next tube. To further prevent a change in analytes, the correct order of draw should be used. EDTA or heparin can increase prothrombin time (PT) and activated partial thromboplastin time (APTT) test results if they are drawn before the citrate tube. EDTA contamination can also give a high potassium. This is the reason the heparin tube is drawn before the EDTA tube.

Certain specimens require chilling immediately after collection. This is done by placing the specimen into ice as you withdraw it from the evacuated tube holder. Any delay in icing the specimen alters test results. The longer the delay, the greater the change. Examples of common tests requiring chilling of the specimen are as follows:

1. Ammonia.
2. Catecholamines.
3. Gastrin.
4. Lactic acid.
5. Parathyroid hormone (PTH).
6. pH/blood gas.

The phlebotomist is not the only person responsible for affecting test results. The patient can knowingly or unknowingly alter the results by certain actions. Patients often say they have had nothing to eat or drink when they have had a cup of coffee. The patient is often under the misconception that black coffee without sugar is not a problem. But coffee and smoking affect the metabolism and can affect the test results.

Exercise can also alter a patient's results. Strenuous short-term exercise can make the heart work harder and increase the heart enzymes. Long-term exercise by highly trained runners can develop into runner's anemia. Stress can have a similar effect—for example, the stress of being in the hospital or the stress of dealing with a disease. In children, prolonged violent crying before a specimen is collected can raise the white blood cell (WBC) count and glucose level count up to 146 percent for up to one hour.

For a detailed listing of specific laboratory tests and what causes changes, refer to the appendix.

URINE, SEMEN, AND CULTURE COLLECTION

Procedures and standards for the collection of specimens other than blood are often ignored because the patient is doing the collection. But even more time should be spent discussing these procedures with the patient so the best possible specimen may be obtained. Without this instruction the results vary, depending on how the patient collected the specimen. Urine specimens have been delivered in everything from butter tubs to soda bottles. Residue from unclean containers can alter results dramatically. Patient cooperation is needed for any specimen to be accurate. Patient education is necessary so the proper specimen is collected and a noncontaminated specimen is tested.

The phlebotomist who works in a clinic or outpatient facility is also often responsible for a variety of patient specimens besides blood. Urine is the most common specimen the patient needs to collect. The laboratory should provide the collection container to ensure cleanliness. For specimens that will be used for culture, the container must be sterile. The urine specimen can consist of a random specimen, first morning or 8-hour specimen, double-voided specimen, timed specimen, or 24-hour specimen. All specimens except the 24-hour collection are best collected as a cleancatch midstream urine. At times the specimen needs to be collected with a catheter by a qualified associate. Collection by the patient is the most common method.

The random specimen can be collected at any time during a 24-hour period. The patient voids in a collection container at the time the specimen is needed. The first morning or 8-hour specimen is collected when the patient first arises from a night's sleep. This urine is the most concentrated and represents a specimen reflecting the patient's recumbent position. The 8-hour specimen is reserved for night workers or individuals who sleep during the day. This still represents a specimen that was collected after the patient was 8 hours recumbent. The double-voided specimen is used to test an analyte at two specific times. The patient collects a urine sample and then drinks 200 ml of water. The urine is allowed to accumulate in the bladder for a specified time, and then a second specimen is collected. Both specimens are tested for the analyte, and results are compared.

The timed specimen is collected at a specific time during a 24-hour period or at a time relative to another activity. This may be done 2 hours after a meal. Blood may also be obtained at the same time. The 24-hour specimen takes the most patient cooperation. All specimens over a period of 24 hours must be collected. Certain solutes in the urine exhibit diurnal variations. Catecholamines, 17-hydroxysteroids, and electrolytes are at their lowest concentration in the early morning. They are at their highest at noon or shortly thereafter.

For a 24-hour collection of urine, the patient voids and discards the first morning specimen. All urine including the next morning specimen is then saved. The patient must cooperate and not discard a single specimen. What is difficult for some patients to understand is that if they urinate while defecating without saving the urine, the 24-hour sample is invalid.

For the best patient cooperation, verbal directions and a detailed instruction sheet in the patient's native language should be given to the patient to read and follow. If the patient is unable to read, the instructions should be read to the patient. The proper collection material is given to the patient, and the patient is sent to a secluded area, usually a rest room. The instructions used depend on the gender of the patient and the type of specimen needed.

PROCEDURE 6.3

COLLECTING A CLEANCATCH MIDSTREAM URINE SPECIMEN: MALE

Principle:

Properly and safely collect a urine specimen from a male patient. The specimen is a cleancatch specimen taken from the midstream of the urine.

Materials:

Gloves
Hand disinfectant
Sterile urine container
Antiseptic wipes
Label and requisition

Procedure:

1. Wash hands carefully using soap and water.
2. Using one of the antiseptic wipes, cleanse the glans (tip) of the penis. If you are not circumcised, this is done while holding the foreskin back. Clean the area around the opening completely. Discard the wipe.
3. Following the first cleansing, wipe thoroughly using the second antiseptic wipe, while maintaining the foreskin in a retracted position. Discard the wipe.
4. Void a small amount of urine in the toilet bowl.
5. Continue to void and collect the urine in the cup. Do not touch the specimen cup on the inside or touch your body or clothing to it.
6. Place the lid carefully onto the specimen container. Screw the lid on tightly to prevent leakage.
7. Give the urine to the laboratory associate.

PROCEDURE 6.4

COLLECTING A CLEANCATCH MIDSTREAM URINE SPECIMEN: FEMALE

Principle:

Properly and safely collect a urine specimen from a female patient. The specimen is a cleancatch specimen taken from the midstream of the urine.

Materials:

Gloves
Hand disinfectant
Sterile urine container
Antiseptic wipes
Label and requisition

Procedure:

1. Wash hands carefully using soap and water.
2. Remove underclothing.
3. Sit comfortably on the toilet seat and swing one knee to the side as far as you can.
4. Spread labia with one hand and continue to keep them apart.
5. Clean labia. Be sure to cleanse well before you collect the specimen.
   a. Using one of the antiseptic wipes, wipe from the front of your body toward the back. Clean between the folds of the skin as carefully as you can. Discard the wipe.
   b. Using the second antiseptic wipe, clean the area again using a front-to-back motion. Discard the wipe.
6. Pass a small amount of urine in the toilet bowl.
7. Continue to void and collect the urine in the cup. Do not touch the specimen cup on the inside or touch your body or clothing to it.
8. Place the lid carefully onto the specimen container. Screw the lid on tightly to prevent leakage.
9. Give the urine to the laboratory associate.

PROCEDURE 6.5

COLLECTING A BAGGED URINE SPECIMEN FROM CHILDREN

Principle:

A urine bag with an adhesive seal is used to collect urine from children who do not yet have the control to urinate in a container (Figure 6.8). A bagged urine collection is used to perform urinalysis or a urine culture on the patient. For specimens that will be used for culture, the container must be sterile.

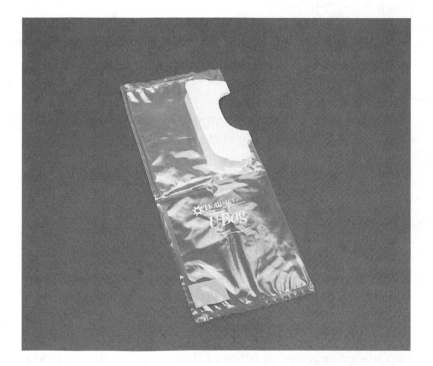

Figure 6.8 *Pediatric urine collection bag. Note. From* Comprehensive Medical Assisting, Administrative and Clinical Competencies *(p. 867), by W. Lindh, M. S. Pooler, D. C. Tamparo, and J. U. Cerrato, 1998, Albany, NY: Delmar Publishers. Copyright 1998 by Delmar Publishers. Reprinted with permission.*

continues

PROCEDURE 6.5 *continued*

Materials:

Gloves
Hand disinfectant
Sterile pediatric urine container
Antiseptic wipes
Label and requisition

Procedure:

1. Remove urine bag from the packaging.
2. Clean the front of the body with an antiseptic wipe. Discard the wipe.
3. Allow skin surface to dry.
4. Attach the bag to the front of the child with the adhesive. Be certain that the urine will collect into the bag and not leak out around the adhesive area.
5. Do not fold or roll the bag while placing the diaper back on the child.
6. Wait until the child has urinated.
7. Carefully remove the bag, keeping the urine in the bottom of the bag.
8. Place the urine bag into another sealing container or bag, and send it to the laboratory.

PROCEDURE 6.6

COLLECTING A 24-HOUR URINE SPECIMEN

Principle:

A 24-hour urine collection is used to determine the 24-hour distribution of certain urine chemical output. Certain solutes exhibit diurnal variations, being higher or lower at different times of the 24-hour period. A complete 24-hour cycle shows the distribution of these variations in the total collection. Due to the length of time the urine must be collected, a preservative may need to be added before collection, or refrigeration of the specimen may be necessary.

Materials:

Gloves
Hand disinfectant

continues

PROCEDURE 6.6 *continued*

24-hour urine container
Antiseptic wipes
Additives for urine preservation
Label and requisition

Procedure:

1. Obtain a 24-hour specimen container from the laboratory. Be careful not to touch or spill any additive that may have been placed in the container before collection.
2. Void and discard the first morning urine specimen, and record the time.
3. Collect all urine voided during the next 24 hours. Urine should be refrigerated or kept in a cool place throughout the collection period.
4. At exactly the same time the following morning, void completely and add this specimen to the container.
5. Deliver the specimen to the laboratory the morning the collection was stopped. The laboratory associate will ask your name, height, weight, and the time the test was started and stopped.

Delay of Testing

When urine testing is delayed for more than one hour after the specimen is collected, special precautions must be taken. This is necessary to avoid deterioration of chemical and cellular elements in the urine or the multiplication of bacteria. The multiplication of bacteria will cause a decrease in the urine glucose. The organisms will also cause a change in pH, affecting all cellular elements present.

Refrigeration at 5°C is often the only method to preserve the urine for routine analysis. Chemical preservatives are used as an alternative in most 24-hour urines and urine that cannot be refrigerated. Some excellent preservatives are found in urine collection kits. These kits provide a cleansing towelette for the patient and a sterile urine collection cup. The patient places the screw cap onto the urine collection cup after voiding. Within the cap is a needle device that can puncture a special evacuated tube. The evacuated tube contains a preservative for either culture or routine urinalysis. The tubes are filled by the technician without removing the urine collection cup cap, therefore avoiding spillage of urine. The tubes can then be sent to the appropriate laboratory with the urine preserved immediately after collection. Preservatives should always be used with caution because the preservative could alter the results of some of the testing performed on the urine.

There is no substitute for the use of fresh urine in routine urine testing. The urine should be tested within one hour. If this cannot be done, the urine should be refrigerated or placed on wet ice so that cooling is immediate.

Semen Collection

Semen specimens determine the number and activity of sperm contained in the semen. This can be done as part of a fertility study. It can also be required as a postvasectomy specimen to determine if the vasectomy was successful.

PROCEDURE 6.7

COLLECTING A SPECIMEN FOR SEMEN ANALYSIS

Principle:

Properly and safely collect a semen specimen. The specimen is collected by the patient. Time constraints between the time of collection and submission to the laboratory are critical to accurately determine the number and activity of sperm that might be contained in the semen.

Materials:

Gloves
Hand disinfectant
Sterile collection container
Self-sealing bag
Label and requisition

Procedure:

1. Collect the specimen after a three-day period of sexual abstinence.
2. Arrange the collection so the specimen can be delivered to the laboratory at a time the laboratory is able to accept the specimen.
3. Do not use any container for collection other than the container you were given when you received these instructions.
4. The semen may be collected at home. Place it directly in the container you were given. Do not use any other container. Place container in self-sealing bag.

continues

PROCEDURE 6.7   *continued*

5. Masturbation is the preferred method of collection. Condoms often contain lubricants and powders that are injurious to the sperm. They should not be used for collection.
6. After the specimen is obtained, it is important to deliver it to the laboratory within one hour and to protect it from any extremes of temperature. Placing the container in a shirt or pants pocket generally ensures the proper temperature. Inform the laboratory associate as of the exact time of collection.

Culture Collection

A phlebotomist working in a clinic or outpatient setting may be involved in the collection of various types of culture collection. Urine cultures are collected in the same manner as a midstream urine collection. The specimen container must be sterile for the culture to be accurate. The urine specimen for culture must be less than an hour old for the most accurate results. If it is impossible to sample the specimen within an hour, the specimen must be refrigerated. Urine containers are available that eliminate this time variable. The urine is collected by the patient, and then part of the urine is transferred to an evacuated tube that contains a preservative. This specimen can then be cultured several hours later with results consistent with a fresh specimen.

The phlebotomist also may collect throat cultures. A patient has a sore throat, and the physician wants a culture. A swab is used to collect the specimen for culture. Commercial collection sets that contain swabs and transport (holding) media are the collection methods of choice.

PROCEDURE 6.8

COLLECTING A THROAT CULTURE SPECIMEN

Principle:

Properly and safely collect a throat specimen. The procedure is used to obtain secretions from the nasopharynx and tonsillar area to incubate for means of identifying a pathogenic organism.

continues

Materials:

Gloves
Hand disinfectant
Tongue depressor
Commercial culture tube with applicator swab
Label and requisition form

Procedure:

1. Assemble equipment consisting of a commercial collection set and a tongue blade.
2. Use a tongue blade to hold the tongue down. Using the swab, take the specimen directly from the back of the throat. Be careful not to touch the tongue, cheeks, or teeth at any time during or after collection (Figure 6.9A).
3. The throat should be swabbed with enough force to remove organisms adhering to the throat membrane. Especially swab any white patches for optimum streptococcal isolation.
4. The collection swab is inserted back into the swab holder, and the swab is placed in contact with the transport media (Figure 6.9B).

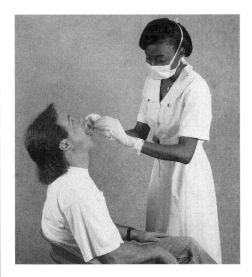
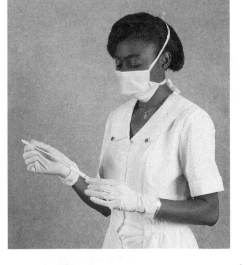

Figure 6.9A *Using a tongue blade to hold the tongue down, take the specimen directly from the back of the throat. Note. From* Comprehensive Medical Assisting, Administrative and Clinical Competencies *(p. 735), by W. Lindh, M. S. Pooler, D. C. Tamparo, and J. U. Cerrato, 1998, Albany, NY: Delmar Publishers. Copyright 1998 by Delmar Publishers. Reprinted with permission.*

Figure 6.9B *Insert the collection swab back into the swab holder. Note. From* Comprehensive Medical Assisting, Administrative and Clinical Competencies *(p. 735), by W. Lindh, M. S. Pooler, D. C. Tamparo, and J. U. Cerrato, 1998, Albany, NY: Delmar Publishers. Copyright 1998 by Delmar Publishers. Reprinted with permission.*

SPECIMEN PRESERVATION AND TRANSPORT

Once specimens have been collected, they must be transported to the laboratory within the facility or to a laboratory possibly hundreds of miles away. Any transportation within the facility is usually done by the phlebotomist or a transporter. There is little time lost and minimal chance for breakage of the specimen. The primary container is the container the specimen was collected in. When a specimen is transported, this primary container must be placed in a secondary container so any leakage or breakage of the primary container is contained. A plastic zip-lock bag is sufficient as the secondary container for most specimens. A single specimen can be placed in the bag, and then the bag sealed shut. For large numbers of specimens, the specimens can be placed in racks to avoid spillage or breakage, and the entire rack placed in a leakproof box. Standard camping coolers come in various sizes and are excellent for this purpose. Whatever secondary container is used, the biohazard emblem must be attached (Figure 6.10).

Some institutions have pneumatic tube systems or robots to transport specimens. This type of transport is more traumatic to the specimen than hand carrying but has the advantage of faster delivery. To prevent the trauma to the specimen, the specimen is

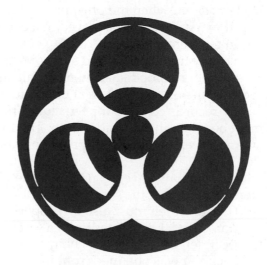

Figure 6.10 *Biohazard emblem.*

placed into a padded container. The tubes are arranged so one tube does not rub or hit against the other. Bags of ice can also be added to the container to maintain the integrity of the specimen.

Transporting of specimens long distance requires more precautions because there can be no leakage of the specimen outside the packaging. The primary container is wrapped in absorbent package material and placed in a secondary container. The absorbent material must be sufficient to absorb the entire contents of the primary container. This secondary container is then placed in a shipping container. The shipping container is labeled with the biohazard emblem and wording that the container holds an **etiologic agent.** Some transportation services do not handle etiologic agents. Check with the transportation service before shipping any specimens.

The integrity of the specimen must be maintained during shipment. Extreme variation in temperature must be avoided. The maximum time the specimen takes to arrive at the destination must be determined. Then the appropriate amount of dry ice or insulation must be added to protect the specimen. All serum and plasma specimens should be removed from the cells before transporting.

Temperature extremes are considered when sending specimens long distances but often ignored for short distance. This is often the case when a phlebotomist is collecting specimens at different nursing homes. A specimen is collected and left in the car while the phlebotomist goes into the next nursing home. In the short time it takes to go into the nursing home and draw a patient, the temperature in the car can change dramatically. The specimen can be overheated or frozen when the phlebotomist returns. Any specimen that is left in a car should be placed in a cooler to prevent extremes in temperature.

Transportation of specimens for blood alcohol testing must be given special consideration. Blood specimens for alcohol are collected for medical purposes to help treat the patient. In most states the laboratory records can be subpoenaed, so medicolegal requirements must be taken into consideration. The medicolegal requirements attempt to ensure that the specimen was properly processed.

First the patient must have given consent for the test to be collected. The person collecting the sample must have documented training. The specimen must also be properly identified and time of collection noted. On all medicolegal specimens, any transport of that specimen must follow a chain of custody. This certifies that the specimen was obtained from the individual named as the source of the specimen. All individuals who had possession of the specimen before analysis are listed, and the technologist performing the analysis is named. During this process the specimen must be secure to prevent tampering and not exposed to extremes that would alter the results.

REVIEW QUESTIONS

Multiple Choice

Choose the one best answer.

1. The glucose tolerance test is used to help diagnose
   a. heart problems
   b. diabetes
   c. liver function
   d. cancer

2. Which of the following statements concerning bleeding times is not true?
   a. You must touch only the drop of blood with the filter paper, not the skin.
   b. A stopwatch must be started at the same time that the puncture is made.
   c. The purpose of the test is to assess platelet function.
   d. All of the above are true.

3. In which test must alcohol never be used to cleanse the venipuncture site?
   a. blood cultures
   b. HIV test
   c. alcohol
   d. platelet count

4. Which of the following would be the antiseptic(s) of choice for blood culture collection?
   a. 0.5 percent chlorhexidine gluconate
   b. 70 percent isopropyl alcohol
   c. 1–2 percent tincture of iodine
   d. use both 1–2 percent tincture of iodine and 70 percent isopropyl alcohol

5. What is the most convenient specimen for urine culture?
   a. any random specimen
   b. a catheterized specimen
   c. a cleancatch midstream urine specimen
   d. a specimen from an ostomy bag

Critical Thinking

1. A phlebotomist is to collect a postdose level of blood on a patient at 1030. The phlebotomist is delayed in the collection, collecting the sample at 1100. To hide the fact he was late for the collection, the phlebotomist enters 1030 as the collection time. How will this affect the treatment of the patient?

2. A GTT is being conducted on a patient. One phlebotomist collects the samples using a finger puncture, and the other phlebotomist collects the samples with a venipuncture. How will this cause a problem with the sequential results?

BIBLIOGRAPHY

American Association of Blood Banks. (1996). *Technical methods and procedures of the American Association of Blood Banks.* (12 ed.). Philadelphia: J. B Lippincott.

Blumenfeld, T. A., Turi, G. K, and Blanc, W. A. (1979). Recommended site and depth of newborn heel skin punctures based on anatomical measurements and histopathology," *Lancet,1,* pp. 230–233.

Geller, S. J. (1992, March 3). *Effect of sample collection on laboratory test results.* ASCP Teleconference Series.

Hay, K. (1979). *The making of a blood film.* Designs for Learning. Kettering Medical Center, Dayton, Ohio.

International Technidyne Corp. (1992). *Surgicutt package insert.* Edison, NJ: Author.

Kovanda, B. M. (1998). *Multiskilling: Phelobotomy collection procedures.* Albany, NY: Delmar.

National Committee for Clinical Laboratory Standards. (1985). *Procedures for the domestic handling and transport of diagnostic specimens and etiologic agents* (2nd ed.). Approved Standard. NCCLS Document H5-A2. Villanova, PA: Author.

National Committee for Clinical Laboratory Standards. (1988). *Blood alcohol testing in the clinical laboratory* (2nd ed.). Approved Standard. NCCLS Document T/DM6-P. Villanova, PA: Author.

National Committee for Clinical Laboratory Standards. (1991). *Procedures for the collection of diagnostic blood specimens by skin puncture* (3rd ed.). Approved Standard. NCCLS Document H4-A3. Villanova, PA: Author.

National Committee for Clinical Laboratory Standards. (1998). *Procedures for the collection of diagnostic blood specimens by venipuncture* (4th ed.). Approved Standard. NCCLS Document H3-A4. Villanova, PA: Author.

Peek, G. J, Marsh, H., and Keating, J., et al. (1990). The effects of swabbing the skin on apparent blood ethanol concentration, *Alcohol Alcoholism, 25,* 639–640.

Pittiglo, D. H., and Sacher, R. A. (1987). *Clinical hematology and fundamentals of hemostasis.* Philadelphia: F. A. Davis.

Renner, B. C, Meites, S., and Hayes, J. R. (1990). Optimal sites and depths for skin puncture of infants and children as assessed from anatomical measurements, *Clinical Chemistry, 3,* 547–549.

Report of the Expert Committee on the Diagnosis and Classification of Diabetes Mellitus. (1997). *Diabetes Care, 20,* 1183.

Slockbower, J. M., Blumenfeld, T. A. (1983). *Collection and handling of laboratory specimens.* Philadelphia, J. B. Lippincott.

Chapter 7

CUSTOMER SERVICE

O B J E C T I V E S

After studying this chapter, you should be able to:

1. Know the three expectations to meet quality service.
2. Give types of nonverbal communication.
3. Be able to follow the nine do's and don'ts of customer service.
4. Explain the five different ways a person will approach conflict.

K E Y   T E R M S

Diplomacy	A skill in handling affairs without raising hostility.
Quality Service	Superior professional attention and assistance to our customers' needs.
Receiver	The person who is being given information by a sender.
Sender	The person communicating to someone else through verbal or nonverbal communication.

Customer service is composed of many facets that can either make a customer appreciative of quality service or angry because the customer's entire needs were not met. The phlebotomist who meets the customers needs is the phlebotomist who will be providing the best customer service. Meeting these expectations is difficult to consistently maintain.

The customers the phlebotomist will work with are both external and internal customers. A customer is anyone who your work affects. An external customer for the phlebotomist is the patient. For the phlebotomist, the patient is not the only customer. There are many internal customers. This can be the nurse caring for the patient, the physician, the family of the patient, and so on. Each customer has an interest in what the phlebotomist does. The patient wants a caring, pain-free procedure. The physician wants timely, quality results. The family of the patient wants a caring, quality person taking care of the family member. The family also wants someone who keeps them informed and does not treat them as if they are in the way. How the phlebotomist treats each of these customers will determine the quality of customer service given. The customer wants the phlebotomist to demonstrate the attitude that the customer is the most important concern of the phlebotomist. A simple question to ask yourself is, How would you like to be treated if you were in the same situation? If the phlebotomist would more often put himself or herself in the place of the customer, the customer service would always be **quality service.**

This quality service is the start of a chain of events that leads back to the phlebotomist. This chain is as follows:

1. Phlebotomist is hired to perform the task of collecting blood and non-blood samples.
2. The phlebotomist gives quality service.
3. Customer satisfaction improves.
4. More customers are retained and tell others about the quality service.
5. As the profitability of the company goes up, salaries may rise.
6. More phlebotomists are given jobs due to the increase in customers.
7. The cycle starts again at step 2.

To achieve quality service, the phlebotomist must meet three expectations:

1. Know what the customer wants.
2. Determine whether or not the customer is getting the service.
3. Continuously take action to satisfy the customer.

These three expectations at achieving quality service each relate to one another. The phlebotomist interacts with customers every day and is required to meet the expectations of the patient. Remembering even the smallest courtesy can keep a customer loyal for life.

COMMUNICATION SKILLS

Communication is one of the primary methods of showing the customer that there is an attitude of caring. Improper communication can demonstrate that an attitude of caring is not being communicated, resulting in customer complaints. Proper communication skills can ensure the customer that the customer is the most important person to the phlebotomist. Each customer wants to feel that he or she is the only person the phlebotomist has to care about. For the moments that the phlebotomist is with the customer, the customer can be made to feel he or she is the most important person in the world. To accomplish this, the phlebotomist must have excellent communication skills.

Communication is the sending and receiving of messages. Communication starts with a **sender,** who creates a message, which is then accepted by the **receiver.** The sender begins this communication cycle by creating a message. The message must be created so that the receiver is able to interpret the message. The message is the information that is being communicated. This information can be communicated by (1) speaking, (2) listening, (3) gestures or body language, or (4) writing (words). The receiver must decode the message and then provide feedback to the sender. It is only through this feedback that the sender will know that the message was understood.

This message is made up of both verbal and nonverbal communication. When words are spoken, we have verbal communication. The words must have meaning to carry a message to the receiver. The communication must be in the language that the receiver understands. One person should not speak English when the other person only understands Spanish. This also pertains to the technical nature of the language. Telling a child that he or she needs to "urinate in the cup" will not tell the child what is needed.

The phlebotomist may need to communicate on a level that the child will understand. A more understandable instruction to the child would be for the child to "pee in the cup." This may not be the terminology that would be used for adult instruction, but for a child, it may be the only instruction that is understandable.

Nonverbal communication is a collection of unconscious postures, gestures, eye contact, and facial expressions that accompany verbal communication. This body language is known as *kinesics.* Talking to someone who smiles at you and looks you in the eye is more pleasant than talking to someone who is frowning and looking at something other than the receiver. Eye contact and a smile can help when it is busy and you are working with another customer. You are talking to one customer, and another customer walks into the room; eye contact and a smile to the second customer will let that person know that you recognize that he or she is there. Customers will be much more patient in waiting their turn if you have recognized them. The receiver can detect these nonverbal postures and gestures even when he or she does not see you. A person who is smiling and happy while talking on the telephone can be heard in the sender's tone of voice.

Communication also includes listening. Listening is often difficult to maintain. The phlebotomist may be trying to listen carefully to the patient but is distracted by the fact that several other customers are waiting. People speak at a rate of 100–200 words per minute. People can listen at a rate of 500–600 words per minute. There is extra time when the receiver can be distracted with his or her own thoughts. Active listening requires the listener to follow five steps:

1. Focus.
2. Limit your talking.
3. Don't interrupt.
4. Manage your own thoughts.
5. Listen for feeling, not just words.

The goal of the communication is to create a common understanding between two or more people. This common ground of understanding is affected by each person's frame of reference. The frame of reference consists of a person's

1. Background.
2. Education.
3. Experience.

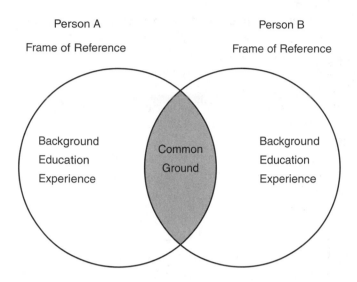

Figure 7.1 *To create a common understanding.*

If people differ in any one of these frames of reference, they may have difficulty communicating with each other. For effective communication, all persons involved must find the common ground (Figure 7.1). If their backgrounds are not the same, certain slang terms should not be used, because one or more people will not understand what is being communicated. Different education levels will mean that the conversation will need to be on a level of the least educated individual. Experience is similar to education, in that the conversation must find the common experience before effective communication can be maintained. There is only a small area that is common for all individuals in the conversation.

Do's and Don'ts of Communication Skills

A phlebotomist can feel he or she is doing everything correct in communication to the customer, but the customer continually complains about poor customer service. The phlebotomist may feel that the customer and the phlebotomist are reaching a common ground, and that the phlebotomist is using proper verbal and nonverbal communication, but the customer is never a happy customer. A slight change in what is communicated to the customer can often leave a totally different impression with the customer. In the book *Customer Service for Dummies: A Reference for the Rest of Us* (Leland & Bailey, 1995), several do's and don'ts are used. Following some do's and don'ts of customer service can make the difference. The do's and don'ts to win loyal customers follow:

1. Don't say: "I don't know."
   Say: "I'll find out."

When you say, "I don't know," your customer often hears, "I don't have the information you want, and I'm not going to go out of my way to get it." By offering to find the answer, even if by doing so means taking a little extra time researching or checking with another department, you score several points with customers for going the extra mile.

2. Don't say: "No."
   Say: "What I can do is. . . ."

Sometimes you have to say no to a customer's request. Rather than using what Leland and Bailey (1995) call a "hard no," where no alternatives are provided, focus on what you can do. Starting your sentence with "What I can do is . . ." shows customers that you are taking a problem-solving approach to their situation.

3. Don't say: "That's not my job."
   Say: "This is who can help you. . . ."

When customers ask you to do something that you don't have the authority or knowledge to carry out, become a catalyst by leading them to the person or department who can help solve the problem.

4. Don't say: "You're right, this stinks."
   Say: "I understand your frustration."

If a customer expresses annoyance at something another person or department has done, do not make matters worse by commiserating with the customer. Instead of agreeing with the negative comment, express empathy by saying, "I understand how frustrating this must be." Empathy is showing care and concern without agreeing or disagreeing with what the customer said.

5. Don't say: "That's not my fault."
   Say: "Let's see what we can do about this."

If an angry customer accuses you of creating a problem, the natural reaction is to become defensive. If you allow this reaction to take over, your mind becomes closed to hearing what the customer has to say. Before you say, "That's not my fault," stop, take a breath, and then, with all the empathy you can muster, say, "Let's see what we can do about this." By resisting the urge to defend yourself, you can resolve the problem faster and with less stress.

6. Don't say: "You need to talk to my manager."
      Say: "I can help you."

Customers sometimes ask you for things that are outside of the facility's policy or procedure. Passing them off to your manager is tempting. Instead, focus on what you can do to help them. If your manager is needed, go to him or her yourself and return to the customer with a solution in hand. This makes you the service hero.

7. Don't say: "You want it by when?"
      Say: "I'll try my best."

When customers demand something that is unreasonable or difficult to provide, your first reaction may be annoyance. Because you have little control over such requests, the best approach is to resist a negative judgment and try your best to accommodate the requests. Do not promise something with the hope that you can deliver. Giving unrealistic expectations may get customers off your back now, but it may blow up later. Make promises you know you can accomplish. Assure customers, with confidence, that their deadline is important and that you will try your best to meet it.

8. Don't say: "Calm down."
      Say: "I'm sorry."

When customers are upset, angry, frustrated or concerned, telling them to calm down is like saying that their feelings don't matter. If you want a customer to calm down, take the opposite approach and apologize. Apologizing does not mean you agree with the customer's point of view, it means that you are sorry for what has happened and the negative impact it has on them.

9. Don't say: "I'm busy right now."
      Say: "I'll be with you in just a moment."

Stopping to assist another customer who is asking for your help is not always easy, especially when you are already helping a customer. Some people handle this by tossing out a curt, "I'm busy right now" at the customer. Stellar service providers use a better approach by saying, "I'll be with you in just a moment." This little sentence, along with a pleasant tone of voice, let's your customers know that you are aware of them and you will help them soon.

CONFLICT MANAGEMENT

In time, the phlebotomist will need to deal with the angry customer. Conflict happens each day in our lives. This is a result of the fact that all people have differences. Conflict can be destructive to the person, the relationship with co-workers, and customer service, if not controlled. Conflict management is a process in which the situation must be analyzed and appropriate action taken. The action the phlebotomist takes depends on past experience and training.

The phlebotomist will approach conflict in one of five ways:

1. *Accommodator.* Smoothing over the conflict is a method of accommodating, to be the peacemaker in the conflict. There is little concern for the conflict or understanding the conflict. The goal of the accommodator is to maintain the peace at whatever cost.

2. *Avoider.* The avoider will ignore the conflict. Postponing the conflict or changing the subject of the conflict are methods the avoider will use to avoid becoming involved in the conflict. Sometimes the avoider will simply walk away and withdraw from a threatening situation.

3. *Collaborator.* The collaborator works to understand the conflict and work out a solution. The collaborator works to resolve the problem and involve all parties in the conflict in the resolution.

4. *Compromiser.* The compromiser works to find a mutually acceptable compromise that partially satisfies all parties. This is usually done through manipulation and domination of the parties in conflict.

5. *Controller.* The controller tries to overpower everyone and dictate what needs to be done for a resolution. The controllers feels this is a win or lose proposition and will do everything possible to win.

One conflict style is not ideal for all situations. Dealing with a conflict will require the phlebotomist to use a blend of all the styles for the best resolution. To resolve the conflict, the phlebotomist must use his or her best communication skills to handle the conflict in a **diplomatic** way. The phlebotomist must first deal with the customer's feelings. Realize that, no matter how minor the issue may seem to you, it is important to the customer. The customer's feelings are involved, and the customer is emotionally concerned. The phlebotomist must listen to what the customer is saying. Listen for the key problem the customer has; this may not be the problem the customer is explaining. A mother may be complaining that the child was hurt during the phlebotomy. She may be angry because all she wanted was some medicine from the physician for her child, and instead the physician ordered laboratory tests. She was after a "quick fix" to the problem, and now it is going to take more time and money than expected.

To find out the true problem, the phlebotomist will have to ask questions. Give feedback to the customer. Summarize to the customer what you are hearing the customer say is the problem. Do not place blame, define the problem in a nonthreatening way. Through this feedback the customer will agree or disagree. This is the only way to find out what the customer wants.

After determining what the customer wants, try to meet their needs. If this is impossible, suggest alternatives. Clearly state your position, and explain why you cannot meet their demand. Share information that you know to inform the customer, but do not share too much. Confidentiality of all other customers must be maintained. Finally, agree on a solution, and follow up to make sure that the solution was achieved.

PATIENT SATISFACTION

Keeping the customer satisfied is the primary role of the phlebotomist. The customer expects and demands a quality encounter in the phlebotomy experience. The customer will tell other customers that the phlebotomist was excellent at drawing blood, very friendly and that the wait was not very long. The patient does not care about the details or the problems of the day; the patient only cares about being treated kindly and fairly and having a quality specimen obtained. Each customer should be treated like a guest in your home. Treat each patient as if he or she is the most important customer you will have that day, and give that customer individualized attention.

Patient satisfaction is affected by factors not always controlled by the phlebotomist. The physical facilities can determine what the customer thinks of the experience. These can be ease of access to the facility, availability of parking, time it takes to get to the facility, and time waiting to be served. These are the elements that make the customer satisfied or dissatisfied if they don't meet the customer's expectations.

The customer can come into the facility dissatisfied. This is a challenge for the phlebotomist to "read" the customer and improve the customer's satisfaction. Factors affecting the customer's satisfaction could be a previous negative experience, personality characteristics, high expectations, or the time the customer allowed for the laboratory visit. If the reality did not match what the customer expected, there will be a negative satisfaction for the customer. For example, a negative expectation for the customer is created if the minimum time it takes for a patient to give the appropriate information and get blood drawn is fifteen minutes but the patient expected the process to be complete in five minutes. For this customer to become satisfied, the customer will need to understand that fifteen minutes is the minimum time, and the customer needs to allow a longer time to get his or her blood drawn. Helping the customer to understand the process will take time communicating with the customer. The more information the customer is given the better the customer will understand how long the process takes. A customer usually does not become concerned about the time it takes if he or she is getting attention during that time.

The phlebotomist will work with many types of customers. The largeness and complexity of the health care environment confuse some. Some customers are very pleasant and rational, while others are angry, not listening to anything that is being explained to them. Most of this anger is not directed at anyone individually; they are angry that they are ill and have lost control over being able to do what they want to do. The illness is dictating their life. They are worried and angry that this illness is taking time and probably will be costly. Some are realizing for the first time that they are mortal and this illness could cause the end of their life. If their life is not ended totally, their accustomed quality of life may be coming to an abrupt end. Understanding these fears and concerns of the customer will allow the phlebotomist to give the quality service the customer demands.

REVIEW QUESTIONS

Multiple Choice
Choose the one best answer.

1. To achieve quality customer service, the phlebotomist must meet what customer needs?
   a. Know the customer by name, determine the tests needed by the customer, know who the patient's physician is.
   b. Know what the customer wants, determine the level of service received, and take action to satisfy the customer.
   c. Know what the customer's insurance will pay for, keep the patient from waiting too long, say as little as possible to the patient.

2. When two people are communicating, they understand each other when they have a common ground of understanding. This common ground is based on three frames of reference.
   a. language, nationality, experience
   b. education, nationality, seniority
   c. background, education, experience

3. The phlebotomist that tends to smooth over a conflict is known as a/an:
   a. accommodator
   b. collaborator
   c. controller

Critical Thinking

1. Through self-analysis, determine what type of person you are when you deal with conflict. Talk to your friends, and determine how they feel you handle conflict. Are the answers different? If they were, what would be the difference?

2. Ask five people to write down their answers to the following six questions:
   a. What is the price of an expensive car?
   b. How long ago did something happen if it happened recently?
   c. The person will be gone "awhile." How long will that person be gone?
   d. The person had "many" dogs. What number of dogs did did they have?
   e. The friend will return in the "near future." When will he return?
   f. The woman was "older." What is her age?

   List the low and the high value for each of the questions. Why are there differences?

BIBLIOGRAPHY

Davis, B.K. (1997). *Phlebotomy: A client-based approach.* Albany, NY: Delmar.

Leland, K. & Bailey, K. (1995). *Customer service for dummies: A reference for the rest of us.* Boston: IDG Books.

Tamparo, C.D., & Lindh, W.Q. (1992): *Therapeutic communications for allied health professions.* Albany, NY: Delmar.

Chapter 8

COMPLIANCE

OBJECTIVES

After studying this chapter, you should be able to:

1. Explain the laws that regulate compliance.
2. Discuss why is it essential that laboratories maintain compliance and follow these laws.

KEY TERMS

Compliance	Compliance is the formalized monitoring of an organization's adherence to laws and regulations.
CPT	*Current Procedural Terminology* manual (2000) listing a coding of procedures and services performed by physicians. Published by the American Medical Association.
HCFA	Health Care Financing Administration.
HHS	Department of Health and Human Services.
ICD-9CM	Codes taken from the *International Classification of Diseases* (1999) that list diagnosis codes for illnesses. Published by the American Medical Association.
Medical Necessity	Service that is reasonable and necessary for the treatment of the patient's illness.
OIG	Office of the Inspector General.

WHAT IS COMPLIANCE?

Compliance is the formalized monitoring of an organization's adherence to laws and regulations. Compliance for the health care industry is required to prevent fraud, abuse, and waste in the clinical laboratory industry while at the same time providing quality service to the customer. Various laws, regulations, and plans have been developed to monitor the laboratory. These laws governing relationships between provider and referral sources are generally known as fraud and abuse laws. This is to ensure that the customer is not being overcharged for testing or charged for testing that was not ordered and that unnecessary testing is not being conducted.

The laboratory should develop a compliance plan to determine how the laboratory will adhere to the guidelines of the **Office of the Inspector General (OIG)** (1998). The plan should establish a culture within the laboratory that promotes prevention, detection, and resolution of instances of conduct that do not conform to the laws. A person within the laboratory should be assigned to the task of Chief Compliance Officer. This person develops the laboratory compliance plan and sees to its adherence. To advise the Compliance Officer, a Compliance Committee should be formed to assist in the implementation of the compliance program. This committee consists of individuals from various responsibilities within the organization.

WHY COMPLIANCE IS ESSENTIAL

Compliance is essential to prevent overcharging to the patient, Medicare, Medicaid, or the insurance carrier. In 1992 a civil false claim case of *United States ex rel Dowden versus National Health Laboratories, Inc.* was settled. This case involved a multimillion dollar settlement between the government and National Health Laboratory. This was the first of several cases involving laboratories. In this case, the laboratory was offering a special chemistry panel to physicians for a set price. This special chemistry panel included the Medicare/Medicaid-approved panel elements but also additional tests that could be billed to Medicare/Medicaid. The traditional chemistry panel that did not have the additional tests added had been eliminated from the laboratory requisition. Physicians ordered the special chemistry panel, thinking that they had ordered the traditional panel. Instead of one bill being sent to Medicare/Medicaid, as was being done with the physician,

Medicare/Medicaid received a bill for the chemistry panel and any additional tests the laboratory added onto the special chemistry panel. In one part of the National Health Laboratory case, the reimbursement from Medicare grew from $500,000 to $31,000,000 in one year. Each patient who had a chemistry panel did not have a **medical necessity** for the additional tests. Therefore Medicare was being charged for tests that were not needed to diagnose or treat the patient.

The government indicated that National Health Laboratory had manipulated the physicians into ordering medically unnecessary tests that had been added to the chemistry panel. These medically unnecessary tests had been fraudulently charged to Medicare while the physicians were not charged an increase. The physician was unaware of the increase in charge to Medicare.

The National Health Laboratory case was the first of several cases that resulted in multimillion-dollar fines. As a result of this government enforcement, the panels approved by the American Medical Association were developed (Chapter 1, Figure 1.2).

LAWS THAT REGULATE COMPLIANCE

The laws that regulate fraud and abuse generally have monetary penalties for noncompliance. Sometimes the penalties are assessed in multiples (e.g., two or three times) the amount originally billed. For some laws the penalty is up to $15,000 per service (laboratory test) billed. Criminal penalties and imprisonment for individuals can occur. Companies may be excluded from participating in Medicare, Medicaid, and other state or federal programs. A general description of the pertinent laws follows.

Antikickback Law

The federal antikickback law prohibits the knowing and willful payment or offer of any remuneration directly or indirectly in return for inducing, referring, or soliciting services including laboratory testing paid for by a federal health program. Remuneration can be anything of service or value. These items of value could include computer equipment, laboratory equipment, or free courtesy testing. The thing of value does not have to be given to the physician. It could be given to an employee or relative of the physician, and it would still be considered a kickback. To test whether the law is violated, the question should be asked: can the service provided to the physician be reasonably deemed to be directly related to the services provided, or does it provide a broader benefit? Examples of fraud follow:

1. A laboratory-provided phlebotomist in the physician office doing duties not related to phlebotomy and normally done by the office staff.
2. Providing disposal of biological wastes that are a result of the physician office and not the laboratory testing.
3. Providing of computers and faxes that are not exclusively used by the laboratory.
4. Professional courtesy testing.

Penalties for violation of the antikickback law are imprisonment up to five years and/or fines up to $25,000. Exclusion from Medicare/Medicaid is possible.

Stark Law

The Stark Law, designed by U.S. Representative Frotney (Pete) Stark, forbids a physician from referring a specimen to a laboratory in which the physician or an immediate family member has a financial interest. The following are prohibited by the Stark Law:

1. The physician refers a Medicare patient to a laboratory and has a financial relationship with the laboratory.
2. The laboratory submits a claim to Medicare or Medicaid for the service provided to a patient whose physician has a financial interest.

Penalties for violation of the Stark law are fines up to $15,000 per service and/or twice the amount originally billed. Exclusion from Medicare/Medicaid is possible.

False Claims Act

The False Claims Act prohibits knowingly presenting a false claim to the government. *Knowingly* is the reckless disregard for the truth. Specific intent to defraud is not required. Examples of false claims are:

1. Billing for services that are not medically necessary for diagnosis or treatment of a Medicare patient.
2. Billing for services not performed.
3. "Upcoding" (misrepresenting the services performed) to increase reimbursement.

4. Filing duplicate claims for the same service.
5. Inserting diagnosis codes that were not provided by the physician.

Penalties for the violation of the False Claims Act include treble damages (three times the amount of the damage sustained by the government) and a mandatory penalty of $5,000–$10,000 per claim. Exclusion from Medicare/Medicaid is possible.

Civil Monetary Penalties Laws

The Civil Monetary Penalties Law applies to claims for services that are not provided as claimed. These false claims are similar to the false claims under the False Claims Act. The penalties can result in fines up to twice the amount billed to the government and up to $10,000 per service. Exclusion from Medicare/Medicaid is possible.

State Laws

Many states have their own set of laws that prohibit the payment of referral fees as well as the referral of the laboratory tests to a laboratory in which the physician has a financial interest. These state laws are not limited to the Medicare and Medicaid programs. They apply to all payers, including insurance companies. Penalties vary depending on the state.

COMPLIANCE PLAN ELEMENTS

The OIG of the **Department of Health and Human Services (HHS)** promotes voluntarily developed and implemented compliance programs for laboratories. The OIG offers guidelines to follow in designing a compliance program (Office of the Inspector General, 1998). Seven elements should be included in the laboratory compliance plan:

Elements of a Laboratory Compliance Plan

1. The development and distribution of written standards of conduct, as well as written policies and procedures that promote the laboratory's commitment to compliance. These standards of conduct should address specific areas of potential fraud, such as marketing schemes, coding issues, and improper claims submissions.

2. The designation of a Chief Compliance Officer and Corporate Compliance Committee responsible for operating and monitoring the compliance program.

3. The development of regular effective training programs for all affected employees.

4. The maintenance of the compliance process to receive complaints in an anonymous manner without fear of retaliation.

5. The development of a system to respond to allegations of improper/illegal activities and appropriate disciplinary action against employees who have violated compliance policies.

6. The use of audits or other evaluation techniques to monitor compliance and assist in the reduction of identified problem areas.

7. The investigation and remediation of identified systematic problems and the development of policies addressing these problems.

These seven elements should be included in the compliance plan in the form of written policies and procedures. The policies and procedures should include sections on the following:

1. *Standards of Conduct.* A standard for all employees that details the policies of the laboratory in relation to fraud, waste and abuse, and adherence to all government regulations.

2. *Medical Necessity.* The ability to order only tests that are appropriate for treatment of the patient.

3. *Billing.* The assurance that all claims submitted to Medicare or other federal health programs are correctly identified as services or tests that were performed. The **CPT** (*Current Procedural Terminology*) (2000) or **ICD-9CM** (*International Classification of Diseases*) (1999) codes are used to identify what was performed. The ICD-9CM is monitored under the direction of the **Health Care Financing Administration (HCFA).**

4. *Reliance on Standing Orders.* The use of a recurring or standing order on a patient is discouraged but not denied. These orders, which continue on the same patient at a recurring (monthly or other periodic time frame) schedule, must be reviewed and updated periodically. This is usually semiannually or annually.

5. *Compliance with Applicable HHS Fraud Alerts.* The OIG will periodically issue fraud alerts, which list activities that raise legal and enforcement issues. These should be reviewed by the Chief Compliance Officer to ensure that the laboratory is in compliance.

6. *Marketing.* The laboratory should have honest, straightforward, fully informative, and nondeceptive marketing.

7. *Prices Charged to Physicians.* The laboratory prices must not provide any inducements to gain a physician's business.

8. *Retention of Records.* All records that could be required by state or federal law are available if the laboratory comes under government scrutiny.

9. *Compliance as an Element of a Performance Plan.* Adherence to compliance must be a part of the evaluation of all employees. The employees must be periodically trained in new compliance policies and procedures.

PHLEBOTOMY-RELATED COMPLIANCE POLICIES

Compliance covers a wide area in the laboratory. Many compliance policies do not relate to the phlebotomist. For the purposes of this text, the policies that directly relate to the phlebotomist are discussed. Laboratory compliance plans require written compliance policies. A three-ring notebook is the best way to keep the policies. As policies change they can be easily removed and a new policy inserted. The policies and information that a phlebotomist should be aware of are discussed next.

Requisition Design

The requisition used by the laboratory should have a standardized listing of tests for the most commonly ordered tests. The requisition should be designed to encourage the physician to order only the tests that are medically necessary and appropriate for each patient. The requisition should include the Medicare-approved profiles and discourage the use of customized profiles that may not be approved by Medicare. If a physician requests customized profiles, the physician must realize that some of the tests on the customized profile may be denied payment by Medicare. All requisitions should include the patient diagnosis to determine the medical necessity of the tests ordered. A physician who orders medically unnecessary tests may be subject to civil penalties.

Client Supplies and Equipment

The laboratory may provide laboratory-related supplies and equipment if these supplies and equipment are used solely for the purpose of collecting and preparing samples for the laboratory to do the testing. Fax machines and computers can be supplied, provided that they are not used for anything other than laboratory work. For example, if a fax machine were placed in a physician's office, and the physician used the fax to send a prescription to the local pharmacy, this would be in violation of compliance. The idea is that, if the fax machine is being used for purposes other than laboratory work, the physician will find that use of value and will be enticed into using the laboratory to keep the fax machine. Computers are the same. A computer could be placed in a physician's office, but that computer could have no other information on it other than laboratory data.

What are subtler are the smaller supply items. If a physician's office draws ten patients a day but asks to be given a box of fifty pairs of gloves per day, then the physician is using the additional 40 pair per day for the office use. This is considered an inducement to the physician to send work to the laboratory. This violates the antikickback laws and could subject all parties to legal penalties.

Courier Services

To get the specimens from the physician's office to the laboratory, a courier service is used and paid for by the laboratory. The physician may ask the courier to transport something that is not a laboratory specimen. This again violates the antikickback laws. The courier could transport additional items, but the physician must be charged a fair market value for the transportation of the item.

Hazardous and Infectious Wastes

The laboratory may dispose of only those hazardous wastes and sharps containers that were generated during the collection of specimens and nothing generated by the physician's office use. The sharps containers can contain only needles used for blood collection and no needles the physician has used to give injections. Any hazardous waste that the laboratory disposes must be old blood tubes and no other items such as bloody dressing changes. The law is working to avoid anything of value—including a service such as hazardous waste disposal—being given to the physician to entice the physician to continue with the laboratory.

Phlebotomy Services

The laboratory may place a phlebotomist in a physician's office to provide specimen collection that is convenient to the patient. The laboratory cannot place a phlebotomist in a physician's office as a cost-cutting measure for the physician. Before the phlebotomist can be placed, the physician and the laboratory must agree that the phlebotomist is being placed there for the sole purpose of collecting specimens for the laboratory.

The phlebotomist is *permitted* to:

1. Obtain specimens from patients when the specimen is sent to the laboratory providing the phlebotomist.
2. Prepare these specimens for shipment to the laboratory.
3. Enter billing or other information on the laboratory patients into a computer system provided by the laboratory.
4. Perform any other functions related to the laboratory specimen collection or testing.

The phlebotomist is *prohibited* from:

1. Taking vital signs or performing other nursing functions not related to the collection of specimens.
2. Filling reports, answering telephones, or performing other functions that are normally done by the physician's staff.
3. Entering billing or performing tests for the physician's office.
4. Reviewing patient's charts for diagnosis information.
5. Performing any duty that is not related to the laboratory and specimen collection.

The phlebotomist in a physician's office is in a unique position and for the first time is permitted to say, "it's not my job." Doing any job that is not related to the collection or shipment of the specimens can put the laboratory in violation of antikickback laws.

Questionable Test Requests

At times a physician will write an order that the phlebotomist cannot interpret, or the requested test was not marked on the requisition. The patient cannot be asked what test the physician ordered or have the patient help read the physician's handwriting. In each of these cases, the phlebotomist will need to contact the physician to clarify what is wanted.

If the diagnosis is not given, the patient cannot be asked, "What is wrong with you?" to determine a diagnosis. A diagnosis cannot be determined from the test that is ordered. If a glucose was ordered, the phlebotomist cannot write down diabetes as a diagnosis. The diagnosis must come from the physician.

A physician will often give a handwritten order that cannot be found in the laboratory list of tests. Such a requested test is nonspecific in that it does not have an exact match to any other test. The phlebotomist cannot assume that the physician wants a specific test without checking with that physician.

Each time that a physician must be called to verify an order or diagnosis, this must be documented.

Documentation Needed When a Physician Is Called to Question an Order

- Time and date of confirmation of the question.
- Any diagnosis information obtained.
- Name of the individual with whom the phlebotomist spoke.
- The initials of the phlebotomist.
- Any instructions given by the physician.

Release of Test Information

The phlebotomist will often be asked to give patient results to someone other than the ordering physician. The results can be released only to the person who ordered the tests. This policy is followed to maintain confidentiality of patient results. The Clinical Laboratory Improvement Act of 1988 (CLIA 88) states that results can be released only to authorized persons or the individual responsible for utilizing patient results. The patient cannot receive his or her own results unless the physician has given permission. This may upset the patient, but the phlebotomist must explain to the patient that the physician has to request that the results be released.

The patient will often go to a specialist and then ask the phlebotomist to have a copy of the results sent to the family physician. Unless the specialist specifically wrote that the results can be released to the family physician, no copy of the result can be sent.

Results can be released to another physician only if a different physician starts treating the patient for an emergency. For example, Joe Smith came in for a complete blood count (CBC) today as an outpatient and then later in the day went to the emergency room for abdominal pain. The emergency physician could request the results of the CBC. The emergency physician was not the ordering physician, but the result could be released to the emergency physician, because that is the physician treating the patient and these results could be critical to the treatment of the patient.

The job of phlebotomy is now a job requiring thought before action. Compliance has restricted the phlebotomist in many tasks that the phlebotomist may be willing to do in order to be helpful. The phlebotomist in the physician's office cannot file records for the physician to help out. Supplies and equipment cannot be given to a physician to make the job easier. All of the restrictions seem at times to be against good customer service. Compliance is good customer service because it helps the customer avoid being overcharged for tests through double billing or unnecessary testing.

REVIEW QUESTIONS

Multiple Choice

Choose the one best answer.

1. The OIG is:
   a. Office of Inspector General
   b. Office of Independent Guidance
   c. Office of International Government

2. Of the three situations listed next, which one is compliant with the antikickback law?
   a. furnishing a computer for the physician to keep his office records on
   b. leasing space in the physician's office, with the physician using half the space for the office manager's office
   c. furnishing the physician with the blood collection tubes that are returned to the furnishing laboratory for testing

3. A patient is having blood collected and asks the phlebotomist to have a copy of the results sent to a physician who was not listed on the requisition. What should the phlebotomist do?
   a. Give the patient the results.
   b. Show the patient the results in the computer but not print out a copy for the patient.
   c. Check the order to see if there was a "release results to the patient" signed by the physician.

Critical Thinking

1. A physician's office draws samples from an average of ten patients a day. The physician's office requests a box of fifty pairs of gloves per day from the laboratory. How would you handle this request?

2. A phlebotomist is placed in a physician's office, and the phlebotomist has a large amount of extra time between draws. The phlebotomist likes to stay busy, so he helps the physician's office staff with checking in patients and filing medical records. Is this phlebotomist putting the laboratory in a possible violation of the antikickback law?

BIBLIOGRAPHY

Office of the Inspector General. (1998, February). OIG's compliance program guidance for hospitals. *Federal Register,* 8987.

American Medical Association (2000) Current Procedural terminology. Chicago: American Medical Association.

American Medical Association (1999) International classification of diseases, clinical modifications. Chicago: American Medical Association.

US Department of Health and Human Services, Health Care Financing Administration. (1992, February 28) Clinical laboratory improvement amendments 1988. (Federal Register No. 069-001-00042-4) Washington, D.C.: U.S. Government Printing Office.

Priest, Dana. Washington Post. December 19, 1992. Lab Firm to pay $110 million in Blood Test Fraud. Page AO1.

Chapter 9

COMPETENCY

O B J E C T I V E S

After studying this chapter, you should be able to:

1. Understand what knowledge and skills are necessary to be competent in phlebotomy.
2. Be able to set up a competency training program and know what to include.

K E Y   T E R M S

Competency   The ability to correctly perform a task according to a standard procedure.

Training of the phlebotomist does not stop with a short course and on-the-job instruction. Each phlebotomist must be proven skilled and competent in performing phlebotomy. A detailed procedure that takes many factors into consideration in performing phlebotomy must be used to document the **competency** of the phlebotomist. The patient's age, the patient's physical and mental condition, and the tests being performed on the patient delineate the skills the phlebotomist needs to perform the task. At all times the comfort and respect of the patient must be of utmost consideration.

A competency program is based on a stepwise training/competency guide that the phlebotomist can progress through at his or her own pace. The ultimate goal is to have the phlebotomist competent in all phlebotomy procedures for all age groups of patients. This will standardize the training so the phlebotomist will feel comfortable working at different sites throughout different laboratories.

A program should consist of an explanation of the procedure, the written procedure, a competency checklist, and the number of different age groups of patients on whom the procedure must be performed. Each phase is completed and then turned into the appropriate supervisor.

The following details information that is to be covered in a competency program.

FREQUENCY OF COMPETENCY DOCUMENTATION

Any personnel performing procedures must undergo initial training on starting the job, an evaluation six months after the hire date, and an annual competency evaluation. After the first year of employment, there must be an annual review of the phlebotomist's skills. The annual review does not have to be as detailed as the initial training evaluation. Each evaluation must clearly indicate what skills were trained, who was being trained, the trainer, and the dates of training. A final supervisor signature must be on the evaluation.

LIMITS ON INVASIVE SPECIMEN COLLECTION PROCEDURES BY PHLEBOTOMISTS

The limits of what procedures a phlebotomist may perform must be stated in the competency program. Procedures that would be normally performed are as follows:

- Routine phlebotomy
- Blood cultures
- Fingersticks
- Heelsticks

- Template bleeding times
- Throat (oropharyngeal) swabbing for patients age three years and older

The following procedures may have limitations on who is allowed to perform them:

- Nasopharyngeal swabbing
- Eye or ear swabbing
- Wound swabbing
- Manipulation or withdrawal of specimens from indwelling catheters (intravenous, arterial, urinary)
- Arterial punctures
- Therapeutic phlebotomy
- Injections
- Tine tests or other skin tests
- Skin scrapings

More experienced phlebotomists perform some of these procedures. Some procedures require the skills of a pathologist or physician.

PATIENT SAFETY

Concern for the patient's safety and comfort is essential in providing excellent customer service. Patients are not going to talk to family and friends about the laboratory tests that were ordered and results sent to the physician. They are going to talk to others about how they were treated; whether the venipuncture hurt; and what side effects, such as bruising, they experienced. The laboratory also wants to assure patients that they are safe and will not develop any diseases from their visit with the laboratory. The same safety concerns apply for the associate. All associates need to know that their own safety in their work environment is a concern. These guidelines must be stressed in the competency training program. They will help to provide for the safety of the patient and phlebotomist.

Fainting or Convulsing Patient

If before or after the venipuncture the patient faints, do not leave the patient. Call for assistance if additional laboratory personnel are available. If the patient is displaying signs of possible fainting, lower the patient's head toward his or her knees/lap while holding the patient in the chair. If the patient is conscious, tell the patient to breath slowly to avoid hyperventilation. If the patient has gone into convulsions, do not try to restrain the patient, but move objects or furniture out of the way to prevent injury. Notify a physician. If you are alone and have access to a telephone in the phlebotomy area, call your emergency contact (another office in the building, emergency department, or 911).

When the patient is fully recovered, move the patient to a place where he or she can lie down with the head lower than the feet. Place cold or wet towels on the patient's forehead or neck. You may give the patient cold water if he or she is conscious and not nauseated. Keep the patient lying down for at least fifteen minutes or until the patient is fully recovered.

For a patient with a known or suspected low blood glucose level, you may administer small amounts (20–25 ml) of orange juice or glucose tolerance beverage until the patient feels better. This technique will improve a low glucose rapidly but will not change a high blood glucose significantly. Contact the patient's physician to explain what happened. The physician may want to see the patient.

For severe reactions—extensive perspiration, convulsions, persistent clamminess, or gray color—or if the patient does not revive in 2–3 minutes, call your emergency contact.

Treatment of Hematoma

A hematoma is the leakage of blood out of a vein during or after venipuncture that causes a bruise. This is caused when the needle nicks the wall of the vein, the needle punctures through the vein during venipuncture, or blood leaks around the needle shaft. A lump can develop immediately or after the patient has left. The size of the lump is an indication of the amount of bleeding that has occurred. As the blood migrates in the tissue toward the skin, the characteristic discoloration or ecchymosis (the black and blue) will appear.

Several techniques to prevent hematomas are as follows:

1. Remove the tourniquet before removing the needle.
2. Apply a small amount of pressure to the area after removal of the needle. Also apply a tight bandage over the gauze or cotton ball.
3. Do not use superficial veins.

4. Puncture only the uppermost wall of the vein. Do not puncture through both sides of the vein.

5. Make sure the needle fully punctures the uppermost wall of the vein. Partial penetration may allow the blood to leak into the tissue surrounding the vein.

6. If there is a possibility that the patient will move during the venipuncture, the phlebotomist should take special care to hold the patient's arm still during the venipuncture. The best method is to have someone else help hold the patient's arm. This is especially important with the pediatric or combative patient.

7. After the venipuncture is performed in the antecubital (bend of the arm) area, do not bend the elbow with the gauze or cotton ball held in the bend of the arm. The clot will often break loose as soon as the arm is extended. It is preferable to hold the arm straight, over the head if possible, with the gauze or cotton pressed gently but firmly over the area of puncture.

Treatment of a hematoma consists of the following:

1. Immediately discontinue the venipuncture if you notice a swelling (lump) under the skin. Apply pressure to the site, and hold this pressure until the bleeding has stopped.

2. Applying ice packs wrapped in a washcloth or towel will help control bleeding, swelling, discoloration, and pain.

3. The venipuncture site should be bandaged tightly to apply continual pressure.

4. The patient should be informed that a black and blue mark may appear and that it will take at least a week for the mark to totally disappear.

The Obese Patient

The obese patient's veins are often difficult to feel through the layers of tissue. The tourniquet has to be rather tight to exert pressure deep enough to slow the flow of venous blood. Before a venipuncture is attempted, follow the course of the vein. Obese patients have localized tissue globules under their skin that resemble veins when first feeling them, but these "veins" do not continue and will not result in blood return. The median cubital vein is usually the most prominent vein to feel. Blood circulation of these patients may be somewhat poor. Firm palpation is necessary to identify depth and size and to estimate the elasticity and response condition of the vein. If the median cubital vein cannot be located, the veins in the hand and wrist may be more readily accessible.

The Patient with Damaged or Collapsing Veins

Obtaining a blood sample from a patient can be challenging because of the condition of the patient's veins. For example, the veins were damaged and healed improperly. This is usually the result of the patient having been burned, scars on the veins through drug abuse or accidents, or surgical procedures in the areas of the veins. The damage makes the veins inaccessible because the scar tissue is too thick or the vein no longer carries blood. Any site showing damage or injury may inflict pain unnecessarily if used for venipuncture.

Purple or dark-blue discoloration of the skin indicates mild or previous bruises caused by overuse of the site for phlebotomy. Selection of another site is imperative. If no other site is available, insert the needle at a point lower in proximity to the damaged site and thread the needle up to the proper position in the vein.

A collapsing vein is weak, and the vacuum of the syringe or evacuated tubes sucks the walls of the vein together so no blood can flow. The vein refills the instant the vacuum is discontinued. Using a syringe and/or butterfly is the best method to obtain blood from a collapsing vein. The syringe plunger is pulled gently; a light steady pull may prevent the vein from collapsing. If the vein collapses with the light steady pull, a small pull with a hesitation between pulls may be more successful. The timing between the pulls allows the vein to refill. During each pull on the syringe, a small amount of blood enters the syringe. With either method, do not work so slowly that the blood starts to clot in the syringe.

A butterfly and evacuated system works to draw from collapsing veins, but only small (pediatric) tubes can be used. The larger the evacuated tube, the more vacuum in the tube. If a 10-ml tube collapses the vein, draw three 3-ml tubes to obtain a similar volume.

AGE-SPECIFIC CARE

Phlebotomy techniques will vary as the age of the patient changes. The competent phlebotomist recognizes these differences in patients and adjusts techniques appropriately. The phlebotomist works with four age groups. Even though specific ages are listed, there is some overlap in techniques depending on the age and size of the patient.

Infant	Neonate (birth to 28 days)
	Infancy (29 days to 1 year)
Pediatric	Toddler (1–3 years)
	Preschool (3–6 years)
	School age (6–12 years)
Youth–Adult	Adolescence (12–18 years)
	Adult (19–65 years)
Older Adult	Geriatric (65 years and up)

Infant

The microcollection through capillary puncture is the method of choice for the infant. From birth to about 6 months, the heel is the proper area of skin puncture. After 6 months the heel starts to become too thick, and a fingerstick or large toe stick may be appropriate. The choice after 6 months depends on the size of the child. Both of these techniques will require a microcollection of the sample. The puncture must be done with a controlled depth lancet. The optimal depth of puncture for the heel of an infant is 2.4 mm. The optimal depth of puncture of an infant's finger is 1.2–2.2 mm.

The infant's comfort must also be considered in any collection. Excessive crying of the infant can lead to inaccurate results. It is best to be ready to collect the sample before you take the infant into the specimen collection area. The infant should be placed on his or her back for the collection of the blood sample. Never leave an infant unattended; even the most sedate infant can quickly roll off a drawing table.

Pediatric

Venipuncture in children younger than 2 years should be limited to superficial veins. Collection of blood from superficial veins generally is most successful with a butterfly collection set and a 23-gauge needle. Once the needle is in the vein, the flexibility of the tubing allows the child to move slightly while the blood is being collected. The butterfly will also have a "flash" of blood in the tubing when the needle enters the vein. Venous collection can be accomplished with an evacuated system if the child is held very still.

Holding the child properly is the key to any successful blood collection. It is best if the phlebotomist can pair up to draw pediatric patients. Often the parent wants to be involved and should be given the duty of holding the child in the parent's lap. Someone else can hold the child's arm while the phlebotomist then draws the blood. The person drawing the blood needs to stabilize the vein, since children have little muscle tissue.

Youth–Adult

Venipuncture on 12–65-year-old individuals reduces the number of problems the phlebotomist has with other age groups. Individuals in this age group can be communicated to and usually understand and cooperate. They may be a little apprehensive about having their blood drawn. They feel they are in the healthiest time of their lives. The laboratory testing being done may be a realization that they are going to be faced with a challenge and that they may not be as healthy as other individuals they know. They are now feeling unsure and concerned. Polite customer service will go a long way to let them know you are professional and knowledgeable in what you are doing. Each patient must be evaluated for the best method of venipuncture. The evaluation must include questions like the following: Are the veins going to roll? Are the veins small, deep, or near the surface? Generally, the youth–adult veins are supported by more muscle tissue and do not have a tendency to role. Venipuncture with a vacutainer holder is the method of choice for the blood collection.

Older Adult

When approaching elderly patients, you may have to speak more deliberately. Your voice should reflect warmth and friendliness, and your manner should demonstrate your concern. Touch the patient's arm or hand as you confirm the patient identification. Talk to the patient in a friendly and courteous manner. The patient may be unable to hold the arm or hand steady. You may need assistance in holding the patient's hand or arm. You may also find that when patients have reduced or restricted physical function or movement, they will be unable to straighten their arm easily or close their hand.

Observe any unusual physical conditions in these patients, such as thin arms, transparent skin that looks fragile and tearable if touched, and veins that, although easily seen, feel taut and threadlike and could easily roll sideways under the pressure of the needle. Often, the tourniquet can be placed over the sleeve of the patient's clothes to ease the tension and not pinch the patient's skin. Before inserting the needle, anchor it firmly with your finger to prevent it from rolling.

Elderly patients are at more risk for hematomas because of their thin veins. If the phlebotomist takes extra care with the patient during the blood collection procedure, the risk can be minimized. Elderly patients also require extra care due to their slower mental functions. An attitude of compassion rather than condescension will help restore a sense of dignity to the elderly patient.

PHLEBOTOMY PROCEDURES

Procedures that normally are included in the training manual consist of any procedures possibly being done by the phlebotomists. An example of the listing follows:

1. Venipuncture, evacuated tube.
2. Venipuncture, syringe.
3. Venipuncture, butterfly.
4. Blood culture collection by butterfly or other methods.
5. Capillary puncture.
6. Metabolic screen (newborn screen).
7. Template bleeding time.
8. Bagged urine collection.
9. Throat culture collection.
10. Glucose tolerance test.

To complete a compliance program, the phlebotomist must understand the procedures to be followed. The competency program must include an explanation of the procedure, a copy of the procedure, and a detailed observed check-off of the procedure. In a competency training manual, the short explanation of the procedure is in paragraph form, telling about the procedure and the equipment used. This is followed by a detailed procedure in outline form. The procedures are the procedures currently in use, and the explanation is similar to those in the earlier chapters of this text. This is concluded with a competency check-off that is used by the supervisor or designated trainer. The competency check-off is completed as the trainee is observed performing the procedure. The phlebotomist must read each explanation of the procedure and then read through the procedure before attempting any procedure.

An example of the outline of this section of the training manual follows:

1. *Procedure Explanation.* This information is the same information that is in textbooks. The information is a condensed version of chapters of a textbook that explains the principle behind the procedure.

2. *Procedure.* This is a procedure that follows the guidelines published in the National Committee for Clinical Laboratory Standards (NCCLS) (1996a).

3. *Observed Competency Check-Off.* The competency check-off is a form that is used as the supervisor or designated trainer observes the trainee's performance in a procedure. A different check-off is used for each different procedure. Only one check-off is necessary for a procedure. This ensures that the trainee is following all the correct steps of the procedure. An example of the type of check-off to be used is illustrated in Figure 9.1.

PRACTICAL EVALUATION FORM

The practical evaluation helps keep track of the number of procedures the phlebotomist has performed during training. The Practical Evaluation Form is initialed each time a successful phlebotomy procedure is completed. An example of an evaluation form is shown in Figure 9.2.

PHLEBOTOMY COMPETENCY EXAMINATION

The phlebotomy competency examination is to be taken before a phlebotomist is approved to perform independently. The exam consists of as many questions as the supervisor feels are necessary to test the knowledge level of the trainee. Usually 25–50 questions are sufficient. A multiple-choice format is the preferred method of testing. The exam is best taken after or at least before half of the practical evaluation is completed. The phlebotomy competency examination must be completed with at least 80 percent of the answers correct; the supervisor signs off, and the phlebotomist has then completed all requirements for certification. If an 80 percent score on the test is not met, the laboratory must set the standard as to how to proceed. Possible solutions are to have a second test available to be taken the next day or a retraining program for a set period of time and then a retake of the test. The remedial action

Phlebotomy Competency Assessment
Venipuncture Collection

Competency: Demonstrate proper patient identification and specimen collection technique when performing a venipuncture.

Behavior: Patient Identification
Uses appropriate collection tubes
Follows order of draw

Task:	Performed Satisfactorily:
Identifies self and patient correctly	_____
Checks requisition for all pertinent information	_____
Washes hands	_____
Explains procedure to patient	_____
Selects correct tubes and equipment for procedure	_____
Assembles equipment	_____
Positions patient's arm	_____
Ties tourniquet	_____
Locates vein by palpation	_____
Cleanses site and allows to air dry	_____
Puts on gloves	_____
Positions the holder between the thumb and index finger	_____
Uncaps the needle. Inspects needle for defects	_____
Anchors the vein	_____
Positions the needle at the appropriate angle	_____
Inserts the needle bevel up into the vein	_____
Follows order of draw	_____
Changes tubes smoothly; does not move needle	_____
Removes last tube collected from the holder	_____
Releases tourniquet	_____
Covers puncture site with gauze or cotton	_____
Withdraws the needle smoothly	_____
Applies pressure to the puncture site	_____
Disposes of the needle in a sharps container	_____
Inverts tubes with additives several times	_____
Labels tubes	_____
Checks puncture site	_____
Applies bandage	_____
Thanks and releases patient	_____
Disposes of used supplies	_____
Removes gloves and washes hands	_____

Phlebotomist's name: _____ Date: _____

Supervisor/Trainer: _____ Date: _____

Figure 9.1 *Observed competency check-off.*

PRACTICAL EVALUATION FORM
In each box initial and indicate the date completed.
BLOOD COLLECTION (<12 years old)

Vacutainer (5)

Butterfly or Syringe (5)

Fingerstick (5)

Heelstick (5)

Metabolic Screen (2)

BLOOD COLLECTION (12–65 years old)

Vacutainer (5)

Butterfly or Syringe (5)

Fingerstick (5)

Bleeding Time (3)

BLOOD COLLECTION (>65 years old)

Vacutainer (5)

Butterfly or Syringe (5)

Fingerstick (5)

BLOOD CULTURE COLLECTION (ANY AGE GROUP)

Blood Culture Collection (5)

URINE— Bag Technique (<3 years old)

Male or Female (2)

Trainee Name:_____ Supervisor/Trainer:_____

Date Evaluation Completed: _____

Figure 9.2 *Practical evaluation form.*

that is taken with the trainee who does not pass needs to be consistent with all trainees. One trainee cannot receive different treatment from another.

CERTIFICATION

On successful completion of all parts of the training manual, practical evaluation, and written examination, each trainee is awarded a certificate of completion. This is not the certification that is completed by a national testing agency but is a certificate of completion of the competency program for the specific laboratory. The phlebotomist has earned this award and has worked hard to attain this level of experience.

REVIEW QUESTIONS

Multiple Choice

Choose the one best answer.

1. An associate is hired as a phlebotomist and completes the initial training and competency certification. When will the next competency certification be needed?
   a. six months
   b. one year
   c. two years

2. Phlebotomist competency must verify the ability to collect blood samples from what age group?
   a. adults
   b. young adult and geriatrics
   c. all age groups

3. The competency assessment check-off form must include what information?
   a. all the steps involved in completing the procedure
   b. the main steps in a procedure
   c. only a statement stating that the requirements were met

Critical Thinking

1. An associate is hired to do phlebotomy for the laboratory and is ready to work the first hour that he or she steps into the laboratory. What must be done first?

2. An elderly patient comes in to the laboratory to have his blood drawn. He mentions that each time he comes in he gets a bruise. He said when he was younger this never happened. What has changed to make him bruise after a venipuncture?

BIBLIOGRAPHY

National Committee for Clinical Laboratory Standards. (1996a). *Clinical laboratory technical procedure manuals* (3rd ed.). Approved Standard. NCCLS Document GP2-A3. Villanova, PA: Author.

National Committee for Clinical Laboratory Standards. (1996b). *Training verification for laboratory personnel.* Approved Standard. NCCLS Document GP21-A. Villanova, PA: Author.

Appendix

FREQUENTLY ORDERED LABORATORY TESTS

Acid Phosphatase Enzyme of the prostatic gland. Increased in prostatic cancer of the male.

Albumin Major fraction of the five distinct fractions that make up the serum total protein level. Abnormal levels reflect a disease process.

Alkaline Phosphatase Enzyme of bone and liver. Increased in obstructive jaundice and bone cancer.

Amikacin: Predose (Trough); Amikacin: Postdose (Peak) This test determines the concentration of the antibiotic amikacin in various body fluids (usually blood) at a specific time. A blood sample collected five minutes before the antibiotic is given is called the predose specimen and the sample collected after the antibiotic is given is called the postdose specimen. Either sample with a large concentration of the antibiotic may be toxic to the patient. A low concentration of the antibiotic may be inadequate to suppress the growth of the microorganisms.

Ammonia Metabolic waste product normally eliminated from the body via the liver. Increased levels found in hepatic disease or liver failure.

Amylase Enzyme of the pancreas. Increased levels found in pancreatitis.

ANA (Antinuclear Antibody) Fluorescent test that detects the presence of antibodies to several types of antigens present in the nucleus of cells. Different fluorescent patterns and the amount of antibody suggest the presence of certain kinds of autoimmune disease, such as systemic lupus erythematosus (SLE), mixed connective tissue disease, rheumatoid arthritis.

Antibiotic Sensitivity (Antimicrobial Susceptibility) Method of determining whether the bacteria that grew from a specimen source are inhibited by different types of antibiotics. This information is used to determine which antibiotic(s) would be best to use to treat the infection.

APTT (Activated Partial Thromboplastin Time) The APTT finds its widest use in monitoring the use of heparin therapy. Heparin is an immediate-acting anticoagulant that is given by injection or intravenously. Anticoagulants serve to treat or prevent active blood clots. An APTT may also be abnormal in severe clotting factor deficiencies.

Basic Metabolic Panel Consists of sodium, potassium, chloride, carbon dioxide (CO_2), glucose, blood urea nitrogen (BUN), and creatinine.

Bilirubin Metabolic breakdown product of hemoglobin. Increased levels found in red blood cell destruction or in liver disease/obstruction. This test is for adults and for children more than fifteen days old. Neonatal bilirubin is ordered for infants less than fifteen days old.

Bleeding Time The bleeding time is measured by making a standardized incision in the skin and timing the duration of the bleeding. Time is dependent on adequate platelet and vascular function. Thus it may be prolonged in diseases that decrease platelet number, platelet function, or the ability of the vessels to constrict and retract. Often done on patients suspected of having a bleeding problem and also used as a preoperative screening test.

Blood Crossmatch Tests are ordered for specific components needed. Determines the compatibility between donor and recipient.

Blood Crossmatch: Leukocyte-Poor Packed Cells Packed cells with accompanying filter removes 99 percent of white cells. Indicated for patients with febrile reactions or white cell antibodies. Also may be used prophylactically to eliminate the production of white cell antibodies.

Blood Crossmatch: Packed Cells Packed cells are used to carry oxygen to tissues and as mass for volume replacement. This is the product of choice for patients with cardiac disease, chronic anemia, and for those requiring restricted sodium or citrate in liver or kidney disease.

Blood Crossmatch: Washed Packed Cells Washed red cells have approximately 85 percent of the leukocytes and 99 percent of the plasma removed. This product is indicated in patients who experience febrile or allergenic reactions and patients with antibodies to IgA or IgE or other conditions requiring transfusion of red blood cells with minimal amounts of plasma.

Blood Crossmatch: Whole Blood Whole blood provides a source of red blood cells for carrying oxygen to tissues, blood volume expansion, and proteins with coagulation properties. This product is used with blood volume deficit and massive transfusion.

Blood Gases Arterial whole blood analyzed for pH, oxygen, and carbon dioxide content. Abnormal levels reflect respiratory ailments or improper ventilation. Blood gases are normally done on arterial blood.

Blood Product: Fresh Frozen Plasma Fresh frozen plasma is the anticoagulated clear liquid portion of the blood that is separated and frozen within a few hours of whole blood collection. It is a source of coagulation factors.

Blood Product: Platelet Concentrate Platelets are used to treat patients with decreased numbers of platelets (thrombocytopenia) or functionally abnormal platelets. May be useful in selected cases of postoperative bleeding.

Blood Type: ABO and Rh Determines the ABO-Rh antigens present on patient's red blood cells.

Blood Urea Nitrogen (BUN) Protein metabolic waste product formed in the liver and transported by the blood to the kidney for excretion in the urine. Increased in renal disease or renal failure.

Calcium (Ca) Element derived from the diet and present in bone and teeth. Increased levels may reflect hyperparathyroidism, and metastatic bone disease. Decreased levels may reflect hypoparathyroidism or a malabsorption syndrome.

Carcinoembryonic Antigen (CEA) CEA testing can have significant value in monitoring treatment of patients with diagnosed malignancies. Persistent elevation in circulating CEA following treatment or surgery is indicative of acute metastatic or residual disease. Declining CEA value generally indicates a favorable prognosis in treatment of colorectal, breast, lung, prostatic, pancreatic, and ovarian carcinoma. Not recommended as a screening procedure to detect cancer in the general population.

CBC: Complete Blood Count The following parameters are included: white blood cell (WBC) count, red blood cell (RBC) count, hemoglobin (Hgb), hematocrit (Hct), MCV (mean corpuscular volume), MCH (mean corpuscular hemoglobin), MCHC (mean corpuscular hemoglobin concentration), RDW (red cell distribution width), MPV (mean platelet volume), and platelet count. This is an excellent screening test. Individual increases and decreases in the parameters provide the physician with invaluable information relating to the diagnosis and/or prognosis of a disease. Two examples are (1) An increased WBC count is a common nonspecific symptom ranging from the slight elevation that occurs with a sore throat to the extreme elevation found in leukemia. (2) A decreased RBC count may be the result of blood loss, abnormal destruction of blood, or diminished production of blood, all of which may result in anemia.

Cell Count (Cerebral Spinal Fluid) Routine examination of cerebral spinal fluid (CSF) or any type of body fluid consists of a red and white cell count. A spinal fluid should have no red blood cells (RBCs) and less than ten white blood cells (WBCs) per cubic millimeter. Increase in RBCs may indicate hemorrhage. Increase in WBCs may indicate many abnormal conditions such as meningitis, tuberculosis, and encephalitis. Body fluids differ in their normal cell counts. As a general statement, an increased WBC count usually is indicative of some kind of infection, and it is generally caused by bacteria.

Chloride An important negatively charged electrolyte. Chloride has two main bodily functions: to help to control the distribution of water between the cells and blood plasma and to help maintain the acid–base balance in the body.

Cholesterol Fatty compounds (lipids) of the body. Hypercholesterolemia is much-publicized risk factor for coronary artery disease.

Ck Total: Creatine Kinase Enzyme of the heart. Increased following a myocardial infarction. Total creatine kinase is made up of three distinct fractions referred to as isoenzymes.

Cold Agglutinin Titer Measures the approximate amount (titer) of a serum antibody (agglutinin) that only reacts with antigen at room temperatures below body temperature. Cold agglutinin titers may be elevated in mycoplasma pneumonia. Certain viral diseases like infectious mononucleosis, cytomegalic inclusion disease, influenza A and B, and parainfluenza, autoimmune disease, and autoimmune hemolytic anemia cause an elevation of cold agglutinins.

Comprehensive Metabolic Panel Consists of glucose, blood urea nitrogen (BUN), creatinine, sodium, potassium, chloride, calcium, carbon dioxide (CO_2), albumin, total protein, alkaline phosphatase, aspartate aminotransferase (AST), total bilirubin.

Coombs, Direct (Antiglobulin, Direct) Determines the presence of antibodies attached to patient's red cells.

Coombs, Indirect (Antibody Screen) Detects the presence of unexpected antibodies in patient's serum.

Cord Blood (ABO, Rh, Direct Coombs) Determines infant/maternal blood compatibility. If a cord blood specimen is unavailable or unsatisfactory, a heelstick specimen may be used.

Cortisol Principle corticosteroid hormone secreted by the adrenal cortex. Levels of this hormone in blood or urine are used for the evaluation of adrenal or pituitary dysfunction.

Creatinine Metabolic waste product of muscle tissue that is eliminated from the body via the kidneys. Increased in serum in renal disease.

Culture: Acid Fast Method of growing and identifying a certain type of acid-fast bacteria that may be living in the patient and causing an infection. Usually synonymous with culture for tuberculosis.

Culture: Blood Culture Patient's blood is injected into two small bottles containing sterile media. If bacteria are present in the patient's blood, they grow in the media. Identification of the bacteria may help determine cause of fever and chills or other patient symptoms. One of the two bottles collected is an anaerobic bottle for bacteria that cannot grow in the presence of oxygen. An aerobic bottle is also collected for those organisms that require oxygen to grow. The aerobic bottle often contains a resin (ARD: antibiotic removal device). This aerobic bottle contains media and resins that absorb and neutralize antibiotics that may be present in the patient's blood. With these antibiotics neutralized, bacteria inhibited by the antibiotics are able to grow. After the bacteria grow they are identified.

Culture: Colony Count Method for counting how many bacteria are growing in 1 ml of urine. Determines whether the bacteria that are growing are present in large enough numbers to be considered cause of the urinary tract infection.

Culture: Fungus (Mycology) Method of growing and identifying mold and yeast that may be living in the specimen and causing infection in that body site.

Culture: Routine Method of growing bacteria that may be living in the specimen. Both normal and disease-causing bacteria grow and are identified.

Cytomegalovirus (CMV) Cytomegalovirus is a human viral pathogen that belongs to the herpes virus family. This virus causes serious illness in people with AIDS (acquired immune deficiency syndrome), in newborns, and in individuals being treated with immunosuppression therapy. Serologic tests are available to detect CMV-specific IgM (immunoglobulin M) antibody.

Differential: WBC Study and tabulation of at least a hundred WBCs on a stained blood smear. The normal WBCs present are segs, bands, lymphs, monos, basos, and eos. Abnormal and immature forms are also counted. Abnormal red and white cell morphology as well as a platelet estimate are also recorded.

Digoxin (Lanoxin) Drug used in the treatment of heart arrhythmias. Periodic monitoring of its amount in the blood is made to determine the dose to be given. Blood levels too low may be ineffective, and blood levels too high may lead to harmful side effects.

Dilantin (Phenytoin) Level Anticonvulsant drug used especially in the treatment of epilepsy. Periodic monitoring of its amount in the blood is made to determine the dose to be given. Blood levels too low may be ineffective, and those levels too high may lead to harmful side effects.

Electrolytes (Lytes) Group of tests including sodium (Na), potassium (K), chloride (Cl), and dissolved carbon dioxide (CO_2). Relationship among these electrolytes is maintained in careful balance by the function of the kidney, lungs, and endocrine glands.

Epstein-Barr virus (EBV) The Epstein-Barr virus causes an increase in heterophil antibody formation. The presence of heterophil antibodies is highly diagnostic of infectious mononucleosis.

Ferritin Ferritin is the storage form of iron. Anemic conditions associated with increased ferritin levels are megaloblastic and hemolytic anemia. Iron storage disorders such as hemochromatosis and hemosiderosis cause high ferritin levels. Decreased ferritin levels can be seen in iron-deficiency anemia, severe protein deficiency, and patients undergoing hemodialysis.

Fibrinogen Fibrinogen is manufactured in the liver and is used for the production of fibrin. Increased fibrinogen is associated with diseases such as hepatitis, multiple myeloma, cancer, rheumatic fever, tuberculosis, and septicemia. Genetic disorders or severe liver disease can cause decreased fibrinogen. In most cases, decreased fibrinogen is attributed to disseminated intravascular coagulation (DIC) syndrome. This syndrome causes a depletion or decrease of fibrinogen and other clotting factors by overstimulating the coagulation process.

Fluorescent Treponemal Antibody Absorption (FTA) Detects presence of antibodies specific for *Treponema pallidum.* The FTA-ABS test is used to confirm reactive results to a screening test for syphilis (RPR), or to diagnose patients with symptoms of late syphilis. FTA-ABS has been demonstrated to be highly sensitive and specific, but false-positives may occur with pregnancy, SLE (systemic lupus erythematosus), antinuclear antibodies, and abnormal globulins.

Fungal Immune Diffusion (FID) Screening test for the detection of antibodies (in serum or spinal fluid) to the fungi causing histoplasmosis, blastomycosis, coccidiomycosis, and aspergillosis.

Fungus Smear Material from a specimen placed on a glass slide and stained. Any mold or yeast in the specimen may be detected.

Gastrin Gastrin is a hormone produced by specialized cells in the stomach. High levels of gastrin can be supportive of a pancreatic tumor, gastric cancer, or pernicious anemia.

Gentamicin Level: Predose (Trough); Gentamicin Level: Postdose (Peak) This test determines the concentration of the antibiotic gentamicin in various body fluids (usually blood) at a specific time. A blood sample collected five minutes before the antibiotic is given is called the predose specimen, and the sample collected after the antibiotic is given is called the postdose specimen. Either sample having a large concentration of the antibiotic may be toxic to the patient. A low concentration of the antibiotic may be inadequate to suppress the growth of the bacteria.

Glucose Levels are derived from the intake of sugar and maintained by the insulin levels of the body. Glucose is the body's energy source. Low levels may reflect hypoglycemia; high levels may reflect a diabetic condition.

Gram Stain Material from a specimen is placed on a glass slide and stained. The bacteria and body cells present can then be microscopically classified.

HDL (High-Density Lipoprotein) Cholesterol The protein transport molecule for cholesterol as it travels through the blood. High levels of HDL have been correlated with reduced risk for coronary artery disease. Decreased levels may indicate a higher risk for the disease.

Hematocrit The hematocrit is the percentage of red blood cells compared to the amount of plasma in whole blood. A decrease in the hematocrit value can be indicative of destruction of red blood cells, interference in the production of red blood cells, or over-hydration. An increase in hematocrit is the result of an increase in red blood cell production or dehydration.

Hemoglobin Hemoglobin is the main constituent of red blood cells. The primary purpose of the hemoglobin is to carry oxygen from the lungs to the cells and to carry carbon dioxide from the cells to the lungs. A low hemoglobin value indicates various types of anemia.

Hepatic Function Panel Consists of albumin; total and direct bilirubin; alkaline phosphatase (ALP); aspartate aminotransferase (AST), also known as serum glutamic oxaloacetic transaminase (SGOT); and alanine aminotransferase (ALT), also known as serum glutamic pyruvic transaminase (SGPT).

Hepatitis A Virus (HAV) Hepatitis A, also known as infectious hepatitis, is caused by HAV. Hepatitis A can be diagnosed by two antibodies against hepatitis A, IgM (immunoglobulin M) anti-HAV and total anti-HAV.

Hepatitis B Surface Antibody (Anti-HBs) Detects the presence of the antibody to the hepatitis B virus surface antigen. Appearance of the antibody signifies a convalescent state and recovery from the acute phase of the disease. Also indicates prior exposure to the virus through vaccination, or indicates passive acquisition for administration of hyperimmune serum.

Hepatitis B Surface Antigen (HBsAg) Detects the presence of the surface antigen part of the hepatitis B virus in serum.

Human Chorionic Gonadotropin (BETA-HCG) Detects the presence of the beta subunit of human chorionic gonadotropin

(BHCG). BHCG is present in pregnancy, choriocarcinoma, hydatidform mole, and some testicular tumors.

Human Immunodeficiency Virus (HIV-1, HIV-2) Screen Detects the presence of antibody to the retrovirus HIV. Positive results must be confirmed by additional testing. Positive results indicate previous infection with the virus. It cannot be assumed from these results alone that the patient has AIDS or will develop AIDS or related conditions. Negative results do not preclude exposure or infection.

Immunoelectrophoresis Laboratory procedure whereby specific protein fractions in serum or urine are identified in serum or urine by their differing mobilities in an electrical field and by their reactions with specific reagent antibodies.

India Ink Prep Stain used mainly on spinal fluid to detect the capsule on the yeast *Cryptococcus neoformans.* Called a negative stain because the capsule of the yeast appears as a halo against the dark background of ink. *Cryptococcus neoformans* can cause meningitis.

KOH Prep Method of detecting yeast or fragments of mold in specimens such as sputum, skin scrapings, nail and hair, thus determining the cause of an infection in that body site.

LD (LDH: Lactate Dehydrogenase) Enzyme of the liver and heart. Increased following a mycardial infarction or during liver disease. Total lactate dehydrogenase level consists of five distinct fractions referred to as isoenzymes. These isoenzymes may be separated according to their differing mobilities in an electrical field.

Lipase Lipase is an enzyme produced by the pancreas. Increased lipase levels indicate pancreatic damage by pancreatitis and pancreatic cancer.

Lipid Profile A lipid profile consists of measuring levels of cholesterol, triglycerides, high-density lipoproteins (HDL), low-density lipoproteins (LDL), and very low-density lipoproteins (VLDL). The purpose of the lipid profile is to detect disorders of lipid metabolism and to assess the risk of heart disease.

Lithium Drug used in the treatment of psychosis. Periodic monitoring of its amount in the blood is made to determine dosage level. Blood levels too low may be ineffective, and levels too high may lead to harmful side effects.

Magnesium Magnesium is increased in renal dysfunction or failure. Low magnesium levels are usually a result of a chronic dietary or intestinal absorption problem.

Mono Screen Detects a serum antibody that is increased in infectious mononucleosis, cytomegalovirus infections, Burkitt's lymphoma, rheumatoid arthritis, and viral hepatitis.

Neonatal Bilirubin This bilirubin assay monitors neonatal jaundice in neonates (newborns less than fifteen days old). More accurate for neonates than a total bilirubin, which is appropriate for adults and children more than fifteen days old.

Newborn Screen As required by most state laws, newborns are screened for genetic disorders such as phenylketonuria, galactosemia, hypothyroidism, homocystinuria, maple sugar urine disease, and sickle cell anemia.

Occult Blood: Fecal Method of detecting hemoglobin (blood) in a stool specimen. The method detects blood produced from gastointestinal lesions caused by many factors, including ulcers and colorectal cancer.

Osmolality Osmolality (number of dissolved molecules) of serum causes the pituitary gland to secrete, which in turn causes the kidneys to retain, more or less water. Measurement of urine osmolality is a test for the diluting and concentration ability of the kidneys. Urine and serum osmolalities are often ordered together.

Ova and Parasites (O & P) Combination of three methods of wet mount and stains used to detect and identify intestinal parasites or the eggs of the parasite. The usual specimen is feces; however, parasites or eggs can also be found in sputum, urine, blood, or tissue.

Phenobarbital Level Anticonvulsant drug used especially in the treatment of epilepsy. Periodic monitoring of its amount in the blood is made to determine dose. Blood levels too low may be ineffective; levels too high may lead to harmful side effects.

Phosphate (PO$_4$) Phosphorus: Element derived from the diet, present in bones and teeth. Necessary for many metabolic reactions in the body. Abnormal levels may reflect a problem with parathyroid gland function.

Pinworm Exam: Scotch Tape Prep Clear cellophane tape is pressed against the peritoneal region. Any pinworm eggs that are present stick to the tape and are detected when the prep is examined microscopically.

Potassium An increase in potassium is usually attributed to renal failure. Decreased potassium is the result of any disease process that causes diarrhea or severe vomiting.

Pronestyl/Procainamide Drug used in the treatment of heart arrhythmias. Periodic monitoring of its amount in the blood is made to determine the dose to be given. Blood levels too low may be ineffective; levels too high may lead to harmful side effects.

Prostate-Specific Antigen (PSA) PSA is found in normal prostate cells of all males. An increased PSA occurs in prostate cancer.

Protein Electrophoresis Total protein level in serum, urine, or spinal fluid is quantitated, and then the proteins are separated into five distinct fractions based on their movement in an electrical field. Increases in any one fraction may reflect a specific set of disorders.

PT (Prothrombin Time) One of the blood coagulation factors, prothrombin is produced in the liver. Vitamin K is necessary for its production. Test finds its widest use in monitoring the administration of coumadin therapy. Coumadin is a delayed-acting oral anticoagulant that acts to rapidly decrease all the vitamin K-dependent factors. Anticoagulants serve to treat or prevent active blood clots. Protime may be abnormal when there is decreased vitamin K in a poor diet, in severe liver disease, or in some severe clotting factor deficiencies.

Quinidine Level Drug used in the treatment of heart arrhythmias. Periodic monitoring of its amount in the blood determines dose to be given. Blood levels too low may be ineffective; levels too high may lead to harmful side effects.

Reticulocyte Count Reticulocytes (retics) are immature nonnucleated red blood cells (RBCs). Daily about 1 percent of, the RBC population dies, and 1 percent new cells are normally delivered into the bloodstream from the bone marrow. A special staining procedure must be done to count these retics. Retic count is one method of evaluating effective RBC production.

Rheumatoid Arthritis (RA) Factor Detects the presence of an antibody called the rheumatoid factor (RF) in serum or joint fluid. Elevated levels may indicate a diagnosis of rheumatoid arthritis. Low titers may occur in other disease conditions, such as systemic lupus erythematosus, tuberculosis, syphilis, or viral infections.

Rhogam This product is given to Rh-negative individuals exposed to Rh-positive red cells to prevent the formation of Anti-D. Product should be given to Rh-negative women who deliver an Rh-positive or (D positive) infant within 72 hours of delivery. Rh-negative women who abort or miscarry after 12 weeks of gestation should receive a full dose of immune globulin.

RPR (Rapid Plasma Reagin Test) Detects the presence of reagin, a nontreponemal antibody that may occur in syphilis, infectious mononucleosis, malaria, systemic lupus erythematosus, vaccinia, viral pneumonia, pregnancy, autoimmune disease, narcotic addiction, and diseases due to treponemes other than *Treponema pallidum.* A high or rising titer is used to aid in the diagnosis of syphilis. Reactives must be confirmed with an FTA-ABS (fluorescent treponemal antibody, absorbed) test.

Rubella Screen Detects the presence of antibody to the rubella (German measles) virus. Positive test indicates immunity to the virus. If a pregnant woman is not immune, infection with the virus during the first trimester may cause congenital abnormalities, abortion, or stillbirth.

Sedimentation Rate (Sed Rate) Measures the rate, expressed as the number of millimeters per hour, at which the red blood cells settle out of blood when the blood is placed in a vertical tube. An elevated sedimentation rate is a nonspecific response to tissue damage but does precisely reflect the severity of the damage. Its greatest value is in detecting inflammatory process.

SGOT—AST (Aspartate Aminotransferase, Transaminase-OT) Enzyme of the heart and liver. Increased in myocardial infarction or liver disease.

SGPT—ALT (Alanine Aminotransferase, Transaminase-PT) Enzyme of the liver. Increased in hepatitis and liver disease.

Sickle Cell Screen Used to detect levels of hemoglobin S of 10 percent or more. Does not distinguish between sickle cell disease and sickle cell trait. Sickle cell disease is often fatal before adolescence without medical management. Under certain conditions that bring about low oxygen tension, such as surgery, sickle cell trait can result in serious clinical complications. Confirmatory test of hemoglobin electrophoresis should be run not only to distinguish between the disease and the trait, but to rule out other false-positive and false-negative results.

Sodium Sodium primarily controls the distribution of body fluid between intracellular and extracellular fluid.

T-3 (Triiodothyronine); T-4 (Thyroxine) Hormones of the thyroid gland. Abnormal levels reflect increased or decreased thyroid activity.

Teichoic Acid Antibody Detects antibodies to the cell wall teichoic acid of the bacterium *Staphlyococcus aureus*. This test can be used to detect deep-seated staphylococcal infections such as endocarditis, bacteremia, and osteomyelitis, and to monitor therapy.

Theophylline/Aminophylline Drug used in the treatment of asthma. Periodic monitoring of its amount in the blood is made to determine the dose to be given. Blood levels too low may be ineffective; levels too high may lead to harmful side effects.

Throat Step Screen Latex slide agglutination test for the detection of a group A streptococcal antigen directly from throat swabs.

Thyroid Stimulating Hormone (TSH) TSH levels are measured to identify and differentiate primary and secondary hypothyroidism.

Tobramycin Level: Predose (Trough); Tobramycin Level: Postdose (Peak) This test determines the concentration of the antibiotic tobramycin in various body fluids (usually blood) at a specific time. Blood sample collected five minutes before the antibiotic is given is called the predose specimen, and the sample collected after the antibiotic is given is called the postdose specimen. Either sample having a large concentration of the antibiotic may be toxic to the patient. A low concentration of the antibiotic may be inadequate to suppress the growth of the bacteria.

Trichomonas Prep (Wet Mount for Trichomonas) Method for the examination of vaginal or urethral discharge for the presence of the urogenital protozoan *Trichomonas vaginalis.* Identified microscopically by its characteristic shape and movement. If found, a diagnosis of trichomonas infection of the site is confirmed.

Triglyceride Triglyceride is the main form of stored fat in humans. Elevated triglycerides increase the risk of heart disease.

Uric Acid Nucleic acid end product excreted by the kidneys. Increased levels are found in gout, chronic renal disease, leukemia, and various malignant conditions.

Urinalysis and Microscopic Exam Microscopic exam is performed on a urine sample only when the chemical screen yields a positive result for any of the following: protein, blood, nitrite, and leukocyte esterase. Involves noting the different types of cells, microorganisms, and other structures present in a centrifuged sediment.

Urinalysis: Routine Serves as an excellent screening test. Consists of a physical examination and a chemical screen. Physical exam entails recording the color and clarity of the urine. Chemical screen includes the following tests:

Specific gravity: indicator of the concentrating and diluting ability of the kidney

pH: acid–base balance

Protein: indicator of kidney function

Glucose: indicator of carbohydrate metabolism

Ketones: indicator of carbohydrate metabolism

Bilirubin: indicator of liver function

Blood: indicator of kidney function or physical damage

Urobilinogen: indicator of liver function

Nitrite: indicator of urinary tract infection

Leukocyte esterase: indicator of the presence of WBCs

Vancomycin Level: Predose (Trough), Vancomycin Level: Postdose (Peak) This test determines the concentration of the antibiotic vancomycin in various body fluids (usually blood) at a specific time. A blood sample collected five minutes before the antibiotic is given is called the predose specimen, and the sample collected sixty minutes after a sixty-minute infusion of the antibiotic is called the postdose specimen. Either sample having a large concentration of the antibiotic may be toxic to the patient. A low concentration of the antibiotic may be inadequate to suppress the growth of the bacteria.

BIBLIOGRAPHY

Moisio, M. A., Moisio, E. W. (1998). *Understanding laboratory and diagnostic tests.* Albany, NY: Delmar.

GLOSSARY

Additive Any material placed in a tube that maintains or facilitates the integrity and function of the specimen.

Advance Directive Document stipulating the kind of life-prolonging medical care permitted for a patient.

Aliquot Part of the whole specimen that has been taken off for use or storage.

Anticoagulant A chemical substance that prevents the blood from clotting.

Arteriospasm Reflex condition of the artery in response to pain or anxiety.

Autoclave Instrument for sterilizing that uses steam under pressure.

Autogenous Infection Infection from one's own flora.

Biohazard Anything that is potentially hazardous to humans, living organisms, or the environment.

Blood-Borne Pathogen A pathogen that is spread by blood and body fluids containing blood. Typically, the pathogens are hepatitis and human immunodeficiency virus (HIV).

Buffy Coat A layer of cells in an anticoagulant tube of blood that is positioned between the red blood cells and the plasma layers. The buffy coat consists of white blood cells and platelets.

Cannula Device used for access for dialyzing and for blood drawing in kidney patients.

Capillary Action Adhesive molecular forces between liquid and solid materials that draw liquid into a narrow-bore capillary tube.

Category-Specific Isolation Isolation based on the category (strict, respiratory, etc.) of isolation.

Centrifuge An instrument that spins and separates blood into layers depending on the weight of the layer. The heavier elements are pushed to the bottom due to centrifugal force.

Chemical Hazard Any element, chemical compound, or mixture of elements and/or compounds that causes physical or health hazards.

Communicable Disease Disease that is spread from person to person.

Compatible Substances that can be mixed without reacting with one another.

Competency The ability to correctly perform a task according to a standard procedure.

Compliance Compliance is the formalized monitoring of an organization's adherence to laws and regulations.

CPT Current Procedural Terminology manual (2000) listing a coding of procedures and services performed by physicians. Published by the American Medical Association.

Demeanor The outward behavior of an individual.

Diastolic Blood pressure when the heart is at rest.

Diluent Substance used to dilute a product.

Diplomacy A skill in handling affairs without raising hostility.

Disease-Specific Isolation Isolation based on the type of disease infecting the patient.

Diurnal Daily occurrence at a particular time of day.

Edema Abnormal accumulation of fluid in the tissues resulting in swelling.

Endocarditis Infection of the inner membrane layer of the heart.

Erythrocytes Also known as red blood cells.

Esoteric Laboratory tests that are not commonly done. These tests are usually sent to another laboratory that specializes in a specific test.

Ethics Professional code of conduct in treatment of patients.

Etiologic Agent Viable microorganism or its toxin that causes or may cause human disease.

Fasting Having had nothing to eat for at least 8–12 hours.

Fistula Artificial shunt connection done by surgical procedure to fuse the vein and artery together. Used for dialysis only.

Flea Metal rod used for mixing the blood sample that fits inside a capillary tube.

Gestational Diabetes Diabetes during pregnancy.

HCFA Health Care Financing Administration.

Hematoma Leakage of blood out of the vein during or after venipuncture that causes a bruise.

Hemopoiesis Formation of blood cells.

Hemostasis The process of the formation of a blood clot when an injury occurs and then lysing of that blood clot when the injury has been repaired.

HHS Department of Health and Human Services.

ICD-9CM Codes taken from the *International Classification of Diseases* (1999) that list diagnosis codes for illnesses. Published by the American Medical Association. This is monitored under the direction of the Health Care Financing Administration (HCFA).

Interstitial Fluid Fluid located between the cellular components of tissue.

Keloid A fibrous tumor arising from a cut resulting in excessive scar tissue.

Lateral Toward the side of the body.

Latex Allergy An allergy to natural rubber latex. It is an allergy to the latex proteins that are released in the use of latex-containing products.

Leukocytes Also known as white blood cells.

Local Infection An infection affecting only one area of the body.

Lysis The process of cell destruction resulting in nonintact cell structure.

Medial Toward the midline, or middle, of the body.

Medical Necessity Service that is reasonable and necessary for the treatment of the patient's illness.

Nosocomial Infection Infection as a result of a hospital or health facility stay.

NPO Nothing by mouth. From the Latin term *non per os*.

Occluded Blocked, preventing a normal flow of blood.

OIG Office of the Inspector General.

Palpate To search for a vein with a pressure and release touch.

Pathology Study of the nature and cause of disease.

Peak Level (Postdose) A drug level in the blood collected 15–30 minutes after the dosage has been administered or when the highest serum concentration of the drug is expected.

Personal Protective Equipment (PPE) Equipment that is used to protect the health care associate from exposure to blood and body fluids.

Phlebotomy Act or practice of bloodletting as a therapeutic or diagnostic measure.

Plasma Fluid portion of the blood when no clotting has taken place.

Postprandial After a meal.

Quality Service Superior professional attention and assistance to our customers' needs.

Reagent Substance used to detect or measure another substance.

Receiver The person who is being given information by a sender.

Sender The person communicating to someone else through verbal or nonverbal communication.

Septicemia A condition when microorganisms (mainly bacteria) are circulating and multiplying in the patient's blood.

Serum Fluid portion of the blood after clotting has taken place.

Sharps Container Specially labeled puncture-resistant containers for the disposal of sharp items such as needles, scalpels, and syringes.

Systemic Infection An infection affecting the entire body.

Systolic Blood pressure when the heart is fully contracted.

Therapeutic Drug Monitoring (TDM) Collection and testing of blood to evaluate and manage medication therapy effectively and safely.

Therapeutic Range Concentration of medication that is effective and not toxic in client management.

Thioxotropic Separator Gel A gel material capable of forming an interface between the cells and fluid portion of the blood as a result of centrifugation.

Thrombocytes Also known as platelets.

Tourniquet Any constrictor used to facilitate vein prominence.

Trough Level (Predose) A drug level of the blood collected when the lowest serum concentration is expected, which is usually immediately before administrating the next dose.

Vasoconstriction The constriction of vessel(s) that limits the blood flow.

Venipuncture Collection of blood from a vein by penetrating the vein with a needle.

INDEX

293